"

WHAT YOU'RE SUPPOSED TO DO WHEN YOU DON'T LIKE A THING IS CHANGE IT. IF YOU CAN'T CHANGE IT, CHANGE THE WAY YOU THINK ABOUT IT.

MAYA ANGELOU

Many people misinterpret emotional eating only happens when facing negative feelings and problems, but as you will come to discover in this book, even positive feelings, if not managed well, can cause one to overeat and eat mindlessly.

That is why emotional mastery is so important. Not to let emotions dictate how we eat, but eat to shape the feelings which we *want* to feel.

I was once an emotional eater. I know *exactly* how challenging it can be to overcome and not let your emotions get the better of you, tricking you into eating your problems away, only to turn up feeling worse later on.

Why was I an emotional eater?

Because I had extreme low self-esteem since I was about 7 years old. Coming from a mixed heritage of Chinese and Sri Lankan, I stood out like a sore thumb in a Chinese school due to my "odd" English first name (which no pure Chinese person had), my curly rough hair, tanned skin, height, everything. Going to school everyday was like preparing myself for going to war. Whenever anyone spoke ill about my family background, made fun about my looks or even my name, I'd have to put on my defence armour to try and protect my soul from drowning in pain and loneliness.

In the day, I used to curse, put up a tough face, slouched a lot, and physically fought with cruel kids to try and teach them to respect me or leave me in peace. At home when no one was around, food was my sole comfort. Fighting and eating were the only ways I knew how to stay afloat from all the cruelty they threw at me, to not lose hope in life.

Having to face harsh racist criticism almost every day from heartless kids who didn't know better, life seemed bleak at that moment. No one helped me, no one understood my pain, no one was a real friend to me. To make matters worse, my brother was very abusive and had anger management issues. I nearly lost my life in his hands on 3 different occasions.

I felt alone, ugly, useless, unloved. In some dark moments, I even questioned what's the purpose of living.

Reality is, I had no one to help me through my

journey of self-discovery, self-love, and the importance of having a healthy relationship with food through mindfulness.

I've come a long way since my dark childhood and teenage years. Through 11 over years of suffering from low self-esteem and self-hate, now I'm a more confident and resilient person. I became a finalist in two International Beauty pageants in 2013 and 2014, I've found a wonderful husband who loves me as I am, blessed to have a loving baby girl who inspires me to be a better version of myself everyday, and I am an entrepreneur who runs several businesses, one of which is my Life Coaching business, aimed at helping people to overcome their fears and build unshakeable true confidence to create a life they love.

All that I know now about mindful eating, I learned the hard way. What I wish for you, is not to go through the hardships that I did.

I want to use my pain, my experiences to provide you with positive power to build a healthy relationship with food and especially - yourself, in a guided, sustainable way that I myself wish I knew years ago.

All these tips that I'm about to share with you, has not only helped me, but also my countless coaching clients who have turned to me to seek life coaching to overcome anxiety and learn how to master both their emotions and their lives.

If you've read other similar types of books before and tried countless ways to overcome emotional eating but never succeeded at it, I implore you to stop, take a minute, be mindful of your present mindset before proceeding because mindset is key to determining your success.

"Life's battles don't always go
To the stronger or faster man,
But soon or late the man who wins
Is the man WHO THINKS HE CAN!"
- Walter D. Wintle

If you are ready to learn how to overcome emotional eating in a healthy way, to master your emotions, and gain confidence to take control of your life, then this book is for you. I'm truly grateful to be a part of your journey towards a happier life.

Now let's go ahead and stop the mindless binge

eating fiesta that's been robbing you from fully enjoying this beautiful life!

Mindfully yours,
Trish Lee

How to Get the Most Out of This Book

This book is designed to enlighten, entertain, and transform. Where appropriate, I've included thought-provoking questions to spark insight and powerful action challenges to help you implement this material in order to create lasting and meaningful shifts in your life.

If you'd like some extra guidance to build your self-esteem, build up your self-love, and gain better control over your emotions, I've created a free e-book Rock Solid Self-Confidence For Achievers just for you.
Visit trishandco.com/ebook-build-unshakeable-confidence now to download this bonus e-book and find more info.

Remember, reading and understanding something is light-years away from actually doing it. Intellectualizing alone is not enough. I could read a *how-to-write-a-self-help-book* books all day long and understand that I need to have an idea, an outline, a computer, and a printer. But if I don't sit myself down and actually write, that self-help book will never come into existence! Same thing applies to you, dear reader. You must practice being mindful if you really want to be empowered and have a healthy relationship with food.

Though you might be tempted to skip through and only read selected chapters that appeal the most to you, it is advisable to start from the beginning. This will help to give your mind a bigger picture, a deeper understanding into why emotional eating happens and where it comes from.

This book is about using awareness to melt away previously hidden tendencies and behaviors that sabotage your eating habits and health. In my experience, when you become aware of a behavior that's been getting in your way and simply notice it— without judging yourself for what you discover—that behavior melts away on its own.

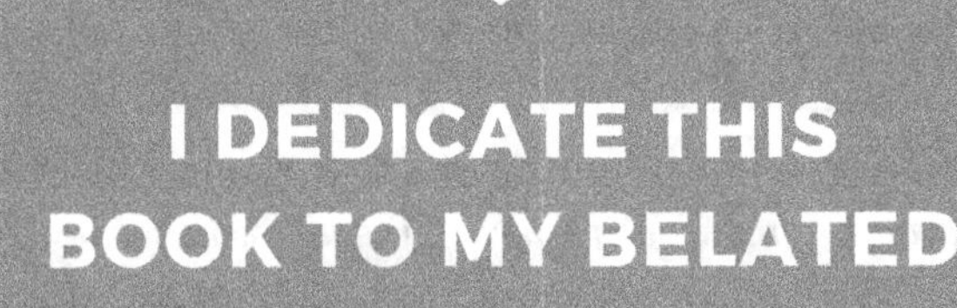

I DEDICATE THIS
BOOK TO MY BELATED

Appa

TERMS OF USE

This publication is designed to provide accurate and authoritative information in regard to the subject matter covered. It is sold with the understanding that the publisher is not engaged in rendering psychological, financial, legal or other professional services. If expert assistance or counseling is needed, the services of a competent professional should be sought.

This is a copyrighted work and Trish Lee reserves all rights in and to the work. Use of this work is subject to these terms. No part of this book may be reproduced in any form or by any electronic or mechanical means, including information storage and retrieval systems, without written permission from the author, except in the case of a reviewer, who may quote brief passages embodied in critical articles or in a review. Trademarked names appear throughout this book. Rather than use a trademark symbol with every occurrence of a trademarked name, names are used in an editorial fashion, with no intention of infringement of the respective owner's trademark. The information in this book is distributed on an "as is" basis, without warranty. Although every precaution has been taken in the preparation of this work, neither the author nor the publisher shall have any liability to any person or entity with respect to any loss or damage caused or alleged to be caused directly or indirectly by the information contained in this book.

CONTENT

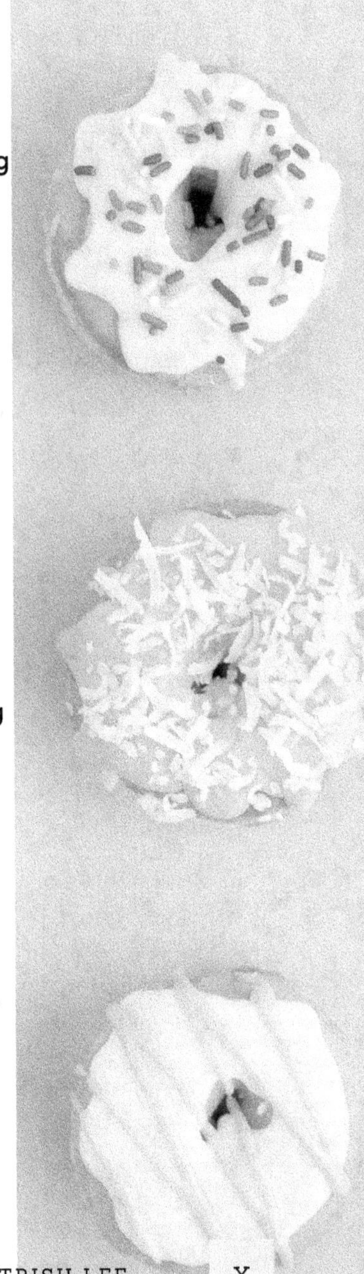

CONTENT

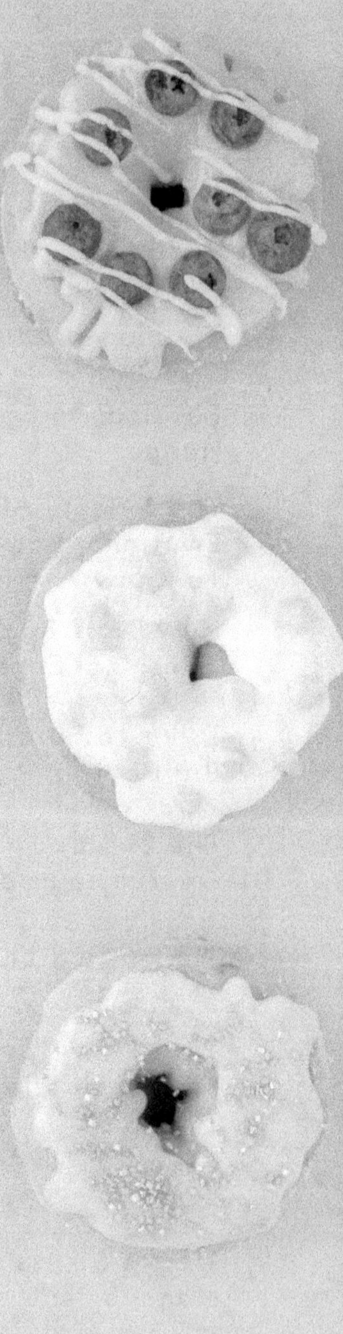

CONTENT

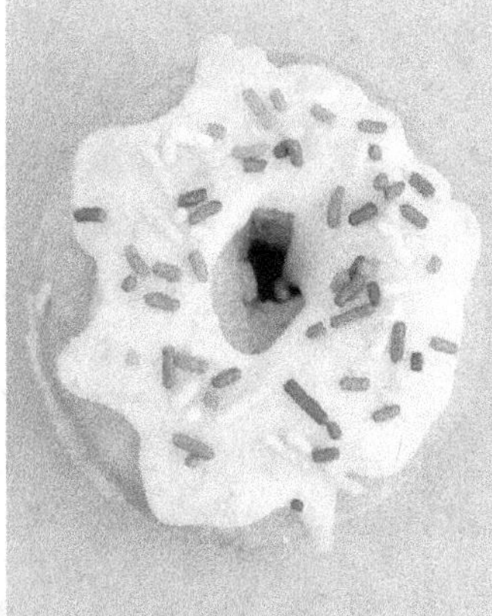

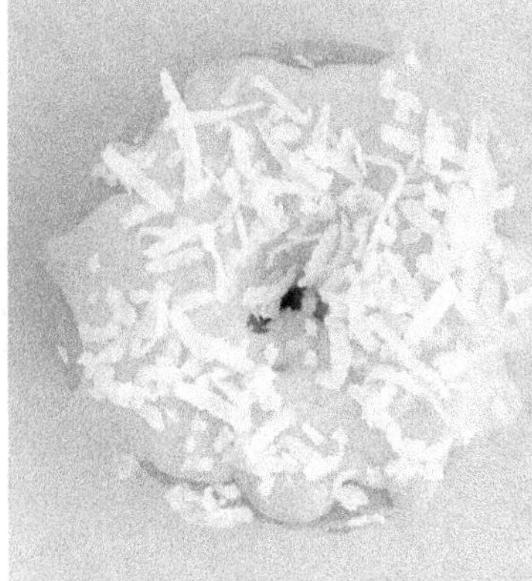

CONNECT WITH ME

facebook.com/trishrlee
instagram.com/trishrlee
twitter.com/trishrlee

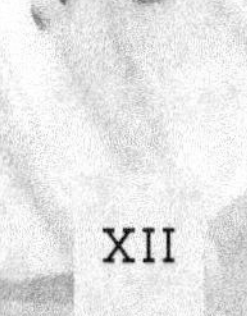

01 | WHAT IS EMOTIONAL EATING?

"

HE WHO HAS HEALTH HAS HOPE, AND HE WHO HAS HOPE HAS EVERYTHING.

ARABIAN PROVERB

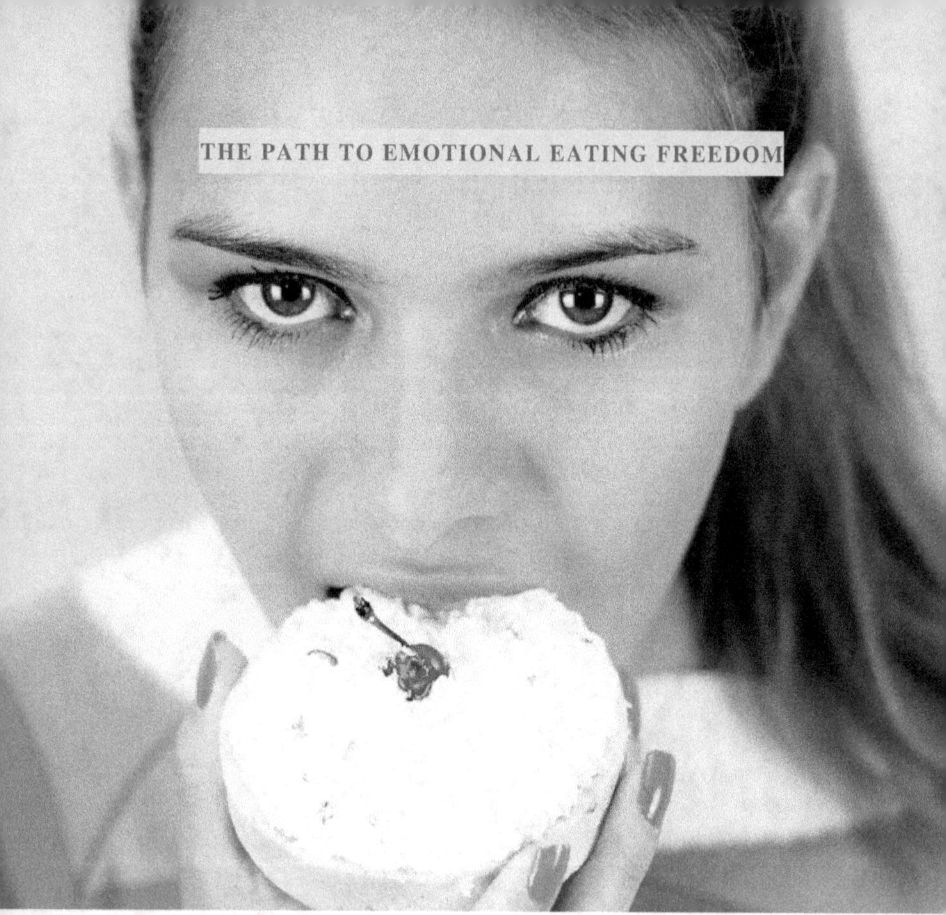

EMOTIONAL EATING: WHAT IS IT?

Do you find yourself racing to the pantry when you're feeling down or otherwise upset? Finding comfort in food is common, and it's part of a practice called emotional eating.

People who emotionally eat reach for food several times a week or more to suppress and soothe negative feelings. They may even feel guilt or shame after eating this way, leading to a cycle of excess eating and associated issues, like weight gain.

Emotional eating is the result of an unhealthy relationship with food. Instead of seeing food as what it is, i.e. something you consume for survival (like water and air), you misconstrue it into something else. You become attached to it, give it emotions, personify it, and make it out to be something it isn't.

Compulsive overeating or compulsive eating, (aka "binge eating"), is an aggravated form of emotional eating.

This was a problem I personally experienced during my teenage years. Compulsive overeating happens when:

1. The original emotional eating issue is not addressed
2. The triggers for emotional eating are aggravated, leading to an increased need to eat to feed the emotion, to use food as an escape from the problem altogether.

Given time, an emotional eater switches from merely eating in response to emotions, to massively overeating in response to emotions over time, since they are unable to get salvation from their original consumption. While not always the case, compulsive overeating often comes with poor body image and low self-esteem.

Emotional and binge eating is more prevalent than you might think. Believe it or not, the American Psychological Association reported in one of their research that 38% of adults say they have overeaten or eaten unhealthy foods in the past month because of stress. Half of these adults (49%) report engaging in these behaviors weekly or more. 33% of adults who report overeating or eating unhealthy foods because of stress say they do so because it helps distract them from stress. 27% of adults say they eat to manage stress and 34% of those who report overeating or eating unhealthy foods because of stress say this behaviour is a habit.

On average in a month, 30% of adults report skipping a meal due to stress. 41% of adults who report skipping a meal due to stress report doing it weekly or more. The majority of adults (67%) who report skipping meals due to stress attribute it to a lack of appetite. 26% say they skipped a meal because they did not have time to eat.

After having overeaten or eaten unhealthy foods, half of adults (49%) report feeling disappointed in themselves, 46% report feeling bad about their bodies and more than one-third (36%) say they feel sluggish or lazy. After skipping meals due to stress, 24% say they feel sluggish or lazy and 22% report being irritable.

Because of how our society has wrapped itself around food, almost all of us have a skewed relationship with food, whether we acknowledge it or not.

07 | 9 SIGNS OF EMOTIONAL EATING

"

YOU HAVE BEEN CRITICIZING YOURSELF FOR YEARS AND IT HASN'T WORKED. TRY APPROVING OF YOURSELF AND SEE WHAT HAPPENS.

LOUISE HAY

1

YOU EAT WHEN YOU ARE STRESSED.

When you have things to do (work / projects / exams), you reach out for food subconsciously.

2

YOU EAT AS A RESPONSE TO YOUR EMOTIONS.

You eat when you feel sad, annoyed, disappointed, angry, lonely, anxious, tired, bored or empty.

3

YOU HAVE TROUBLE LOSING WEIGHT (DUE TO THE WAY YOU EAT).

Even though you want to lose weight and you know the technicalities behind losing weight, you have trouble sticking to your diet.

4

YOUR EATING IS OUT OF CONTROL (YOU CAN'T STOP YOURSELF FROM EATING).

At times you would even go out of the way just to get food or to satisfy a particular craving, even though you may not be hungry at all.

5

YOU EAT WHEN YOU FEEL HAPPY.

You see eating as a necessary companion to happy emotions, just like how people eat to celebrate good news.

6

YOU ARE FASCINATED WITH FOOD.

You love food. You love to eat. When you're not eating, you can't help but think about food. You long and crave for it. When you're eating, it's like you're in wonderland.

7

YOU USE EMOTIONALLY-CHARGED WORDS TO DESCRIBE FOOD / EATING,

like "sinful", "decadent", "guilt-ridden", "love", "lust", "indulgent", "craving", "tempting", etc, even though food is a non-living thing, incapable of feelings nor returning your love or hate.

8

YOU EAT EVEN THOUGH YOU ARE RIGHTFULLY FULL.

No matter how much you eat, no matter how full you feel, you never feel quite satisfied. Whatever satisfaction you get from eating is momentary, and you return to eating after a while to recapture that emotion.

9

YOU THINK OF EATING EVEN THOUGH YOU ARE RIGHTFULLY FULL.

Even after you've had your fill, you continue to think of food. You think about what to eat for the next meal right after you've finished eating. You obsess about X, Y, Z food, and when you can eat it. You can't wait till it's time to eat again. You think about how satisfied you'll be when you finally get to eat.

12 | PHYSICAL VS. EMOTIONAL HUNGER

AWARENESS IS ALL ABOUT RESTORING YOUR FREEDOM TO CHOOSE WHAT YOU WANT INSTEAD OF WHAT YOUR PAST IMPOSES ON YOU.

DEEPAK CHOPRA

PHYSICAL VS. EMOTIONAL HUNGER

It is very easy to mistake emotional hunger for physical hunger. But there are characteristics that distinguish them. Recognizing these subtle differences is the first step towards helping to stop emotional eating patterns.

Does the hunger come on quickly or gradually?
Emotional hunger tends to hit quickly and suddenly and feels urgent. Physical hunger is usually not as urgent or sudden unless it has been a while since a person ate.

Is a food craving for a specific food?
Emotional hunger is usually associated with cravings for junk food or something unhealthy. Someone who is physically hungry will often eat anything, while someone who is emotionally hungry will want something specific, such as fries or a pizza.

Is there such a thing as mindless eating?
Mindless eating is when someone eats without paying attention to or enjoying what they are consuming.

An example is eating an entire container of ice cream while watching television, having not intended to eat that much. This behavior usually happens with emotional eating, not eating due to hunger.

Does the hunger come from the stomach or the head?

Emotional hunger does not originate from the stomach, such as with a rumbling or growling stomach. Emotional hunger tends to start when a person thinks about a craving or wants something specific to eat.

Are there feelings of regret or guilt after emotional eating?

Giving in to a craving, or eating because of stress can cause feelings of regret, shame, or guilt. These responses tend to be associated with emotional hunger.

On the other hand, satisfying a physical hunger is giving the body the nutrients or calories it needs to function and is not associated with negative feelings.

16 | THE 3 FACTS ABOUT EMOTIONAL EATING YOU NEED TO KNOW

"

THE HALLMARK OF SUCCESSFUL PEOPLE IS THAT THEY ARE ALWAYS STRETCHING THEMSELVES TO LEARN NEW THINGS.

CAROL S. DWECK

Fast Facts About Emotional Eating:

✔ There are both **physical and psychological** causes for emotional eating.

✔ Often, emotional eating is triggered by **stress** or other strong emotions.

✔ Using the **right coping strategies** can help a person trying to alleviate even the most severe symptoms.

No matter how long you've been battling with emotional eating, I'm here to tell you that by consistently applying several or all the tips I'm about to share with you, you *can* and *will* overcome it.

19 | HOW DID I BECOME AN EMOTIONAL EATER?

> **THOUGH NOBODY CAN GO BACK AND MAKE A NEW BEGINNING... ANYONE CAN START OVER AND MAKE A NEW ENDING.**

CHICO XAVIER

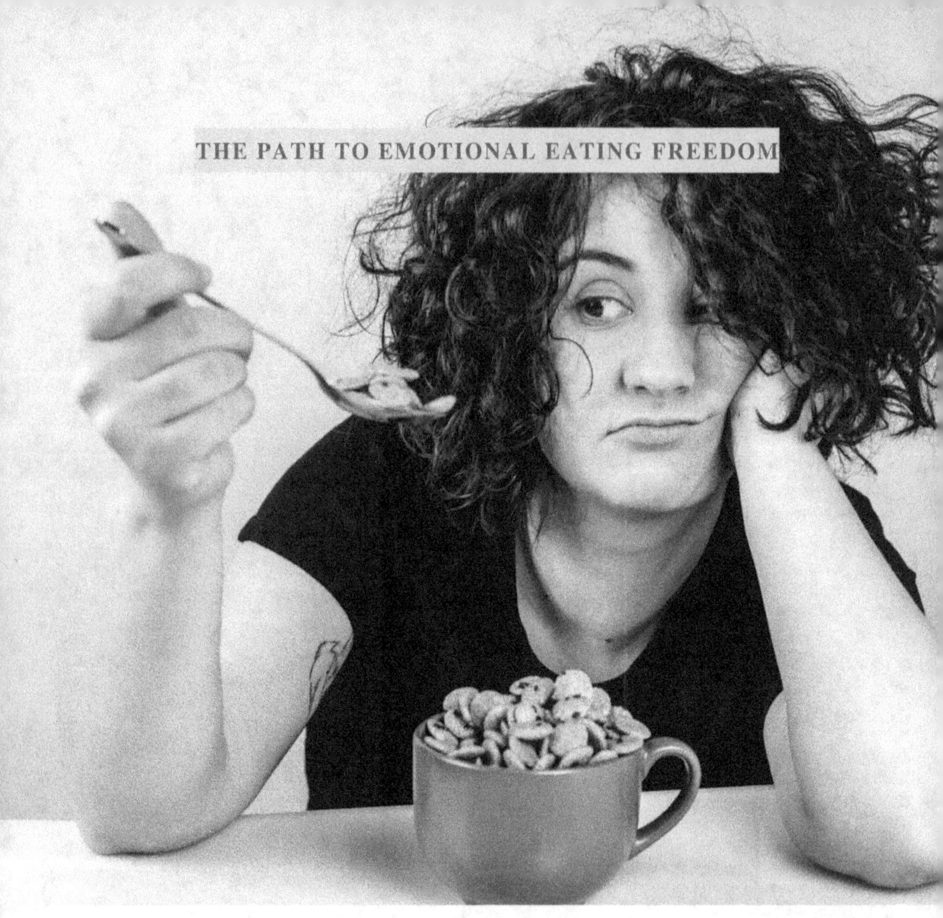

WHY DO I KEEP EATING?

Emotional eating is not simply a matter of a person lacking self-discipline or needing to eat less.

Likewise, people who eat to deal with stress do not just lack self-control. The causes are complex and may involve some of the following:

CHILDHOOD DEVELOPMENT

For some people, emotional eating is a learned behavior.

During childhood, their parents gave them treats to help them deal with a tough day or situation, or as a reward for something good.

Over time, the child who reaches for a cookie after getting a bad grade on a test may become an adult who grabs a box of cookies after a rough day at work.

In an example such as this, the roots of emotional eating are deep, which can make breaking the habit extremely challenging.

DIFFICULTY DEALING WITH EMOTIONS

It is common for people to also struggle with difficult or uncomfortable feelings and emotions. There is an instinct or need to quickly fix or destroy these negative feelings, which can lead to unhealthy behaviors.

On top of that, emotional eating is not only linked to

negative emotions. Eating a lot of candy at a fun Halloween party, or too much on Thanksgiving are examples of eating because of the holiday occasion itself.

PHYSICAL IMPACT OF STRESS

There are also some physical reasons why stress and strong emotions can cause a person to overeat.

➻ High cortisol levels

Initially, stress causes the appetite to decrease so that the body can deal with the situation. If the stress does not let up, another hormone called cortisol is released. Cortisol increases appetite and can cause someone to overeat.

➻ Cravings

High cortisol levels from stress can increase food cravings for sugary or fatty foods. Stress is also associated with increased hunger hormones, which may also contribute to cravings for unhealthy foods.

➻ Sex

Some research shows that women are more likely to use food to deal with stress than men are, while men are more likely than women to smoke or use alcohol.

24 | I LIKE TO EAT... WHAT'S THE BIG DEAL?

"

YOU GAIN STRENGTH, COURAGE, AND CONFIDENCE BY EVERY EXPERIENCE IN WHICH YOU REALLY STOP TO LOOK FEAR IN THE FACE. YOU ARE ABLE TO SAY TO YOURSELF, 'I LIVED THROUGH THIS HORROR. I CAN TAKE THE NEXT THING THAT COMES ALONG.'

ELEANOR ROOSEVELT

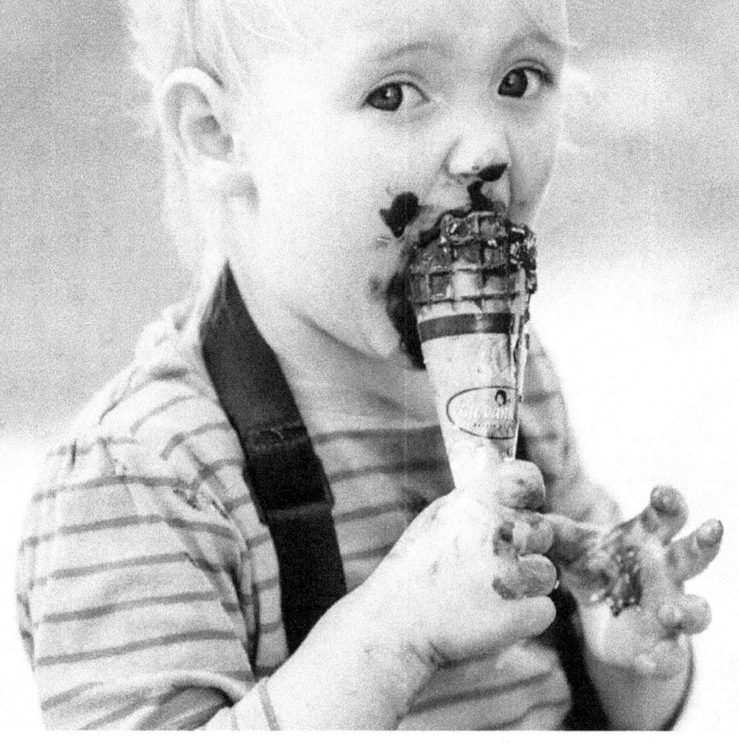

WHY IS EMOTIONAL EATING BAD FOR ME?

Some people might argue that it's perfectly okay to eat in response to an emotion. That if you feel like eating even though you just ate, you should just eat.

If you feel like eating ice cream and chocolate after an argument with your boyfriend, you should just eat. That if you are stressed out and think eating will make you feel better, you should just eat.

I think if you have absolutely no idea how to tackle the situation, and you absolutely need to eat to maintain your sanity at that moment, then go ahead and eat (but try as best as you can to eat in moderation), because I suppose it is the best option you have within the confines of that situation. However as a long term solution, you should definitely look into your emotional eating and learn to address your problems and emotions (or at least develop better stress or problem coping mechanisms in the time being), because emotional eating is *not* a sustainable habit.

In fact, it causes more detriment to you than you can imagine.

HIDDEN IMPLICATIONS OF EMOTIONAL EATING

Say you feel upset all of a sudden. You're not sure how or why, but you know pie will make you feel better. You reach out for a piece of apple pie in the fridge, and you tuck in.

As you eat, you feel happy. You savor the taste of the apple pie in between bites. You think about how wonderful it is to be eating this pie and how lucky you are to be able to consume this food.

And after you are done, you feel all better. With a renewed focus and more positive state of mind, you then get on with your plans for the day.

What's wrong with this scenario?

It may look like nothing's wrong and might well be a common occurrence in your daily life. You might even point out, "Hey! Food has served such a positive role here! What's with all this nonsensical rubbish about emotional eating being bad for you?"

But has it really? Let's take a closer look...

#1. The original triggering reason why you were upset is left unidentified

Sure, your negative feelings were offset by eating. But why did you even feel negative to begin with? Where did the emotion spring from? How long has it been there? What triggered it? And how? Do you even know? Or were you just too preoccupied with the thought of eating, too busy eating and filling yourself in your food, to even care?

#2. Since the trigger is not uncovered, the issue remains unaddressed

Your negative feelings may have been offset by food, but that's only in that instant, and it's merely a surface patch. There is a deeper place where the emotions came from, and that problem source is still there, suppressed among the many other things in your life.

Just like hiding your head in the sand doesn't mean the world doesn't exist, successfully dispelling the emotions via eating doesn't mean the problem has disappeared. It is still there; you just don't know it or choose to be in denial of its existence.

#3. You create a loop in your life

Since the issue is not resolved, it's a matter of time before it recurs, bringing with it the same ugly emotions from before – the ones you tried to use food to erase. And since eating does not solve the problem at all, you create a loop where you experience the same situation over and over, and along with it, the same negative emotions.

To condense it into a simple, linear equation for you:

Problem arises -> Triggers feelings of stress -> You eat to offset stress -> You feel happy for a moment and forget about the problem -> You live on while the original problem remains unresolved -> After a while, the problem recurs -> Feelings of stress are triggered again -> You eat again to offset stress -> You feel happy, for a brief moment -> Problem still does not get resolved -> Cycle continues.

You are stuck with it (both the problem and eating), as long as you turn to eating as the solution, as eating is not a problem-resolution method (that's not what mother nature designed it to do).

#4. You become emotionally dependent on food

As you rely on eating to dispel negative emotions and usher in positive ones, you become dependent on food to make you feel happy. You begin to hanker after food, to dissolve negative emotions when you feel down.

If you are ever denied food when you need it, you

become angsty. Food has become your crutch, where you are unable to function at your full potential when it's not there. It's akin to drug addiction.

While I was resolving my emotional eating issue, I found it very helpful to refer to my friends who have extremely healthy relationships with food. None of them have intentions, urges or inclinations of any kind to eat when they are not hungry or had their fill, no matter how integral food may seem to the occasion (even with birthday cakes at birthday parties).

During the years I was heavily entrapped in my cycle of emotional eating, I thought they were crazy, missing out on life, and were just controlling themselves on the inside. But now I finally realize that it was because there was absolutely no reason for them to eat since they were not hungry, and they were just being at peace with that which is only supposed to fuel their body. There's no control nor discipline to speak of, because there's no urge nor desire to eat to begin with – due to their fully healthy relationship with food.

One just needs to ask oneself the following

questions, to know that there is more than meets the eye: Why is there a need to consume this, when there is no physical need? To derive emotional pleasure, satisfaction? But why would you derive emotional pleasure/satisfaction from consuming this? Why is your happiness dependent on the consumption of food?

And why is it that there are other people who don't experience this, but you do? What is it about your internal wiring that's making you react this way?

What if you can self-generate this same sense of happiness (if not more) by yourself, without food? All of us have the ability to do that – we just lost touch with that because we became emotionally dependent on food to elicit happiness. It's all about reconnecting with that ability in us.

#5. You live in an illusion

You think you are happy, but you aren't. Emotional eating never solves anything, since food cannot fill that which it was never created to fill. The role of food, by design, is to feed our physical bodies and give us energy to live. That's it.

While eating may make you feel better in that one moment, that's because (a) eating food (especially "comfort" food that's high in carbohydrates and sugar) triggers the release of serotonin (a hormone in the brain), which then creates a happy feeling (b) a part of you has been conditioned to link eating with happiness, which makes your happiness a self-fulfilling prophecy.

This means whatever happiness you feel while eating is false, induced, and temporary, as opposed to true happiness which comes from within, without having to eat to induce it.

This also means whatever made you unhappy is still there, floating somewhere in your life. You are just covering it up with makeshift feelings generated from eating. No sooner will that same issue come back to bite you (see point #3) – when you least expect it.

Is this what you deem as living a conscious life? Is this what it means to live in line with your highest truth? I think you deserve better and you are capable of better.

#6. You have to deal with physical implications of eating more than your body needs

By eating out of emotions vs. hunger, you are eating more than your body actually needs, which is unhealthy. This has more implications than you may realize:

1) Weight gain. The most immediate, and the most obvious. When you turn to food for salvation, it's a matter of time before you gain weight – possibly even becoming overweight or obese over time. This is why emotional eaters tend to be overweight and heavier than the average person, though not necessarily so if they exercise excessively to offset their extra food intake.

This is just a temporary fix though (see point #7). Weight gain can be a very traumatic experience, especially if you do not wish to gain weight. It leads to more stress, which makes you eat in response to stress, hence perpetuating the problem.

2) Oftentimes, weight gain leads to a decrease in physical attractiveness, if we benchmark against society's norm for attractiveness. This inadvertently

leads to poor body image, lower self-esteem, and potentially self-hate.

3) Given the food people turn to in times of solace is junk food such as pies, pastries, desserts, chips, candy, fried food (typical "comfort" food), and not salads or fruits, it leads to higher cholesterol, lower stamina, and poorer health overall.

#7. You abuse your body with unnecessary work

This is important enough to be called out as a separate point because maybe you might have not realized this fact. When you over eat, you abuse your body, weighing it down with increased (and most importantly, unnecessary) digestion, food processing, and extra body weight.

You make yourself more fatigued due to all that extra body weight you're carrying around, and you wonder why you're more and more tired nowadays.

For those of you who embark on rigorous exercise thereafter to offset the extra calories you took in, that's additional wear and tear you're making your body go through, when the whole thing could be avoided in the first place via a different coping mechanism.

You may look physically in shape, as if you do not overeat, but that doesn't negate the fact that you are putting your body through work that it doesn't have to go through.

A car that has been pumped with fuel and subsequently had its fuel exhausted via driving around the city for 10,000 times unnecessarily is never going to be in the same condition as a car that is only filled and driven where necessary. The former is going to be in a worse off condition, due to the constant usage, while the latter will be in a fresher condition. It'll be a matter of time before the former breaks down and stops functioning (think early death, disease, heart failure, etc), before the latter does.

Likewise, our physical body does not last forever. It wears out faster or slower, depending on how we treat it.

Do you see what I'm getting at?

The main takeaway here is, as much as good coping strategies can help to reduce mindless eating habits quite substantially, the only way to eliminate it completely is by mustering the courage to tackle the problems which are affecting you either mentally or emotionally.

Once you can solve those issues at its core, moving forward toward a healthier and happy life will become *much* easier.

38 | 21 TIPS TO MINDFULLY OVERCOME EMOTIONAL EATING

> # I LEARNED THAT COURAGE WAS NOT THE ABSENCE OF FEAR, BUT THE TRIUMPH OVER IT. THE BRAVE MAN IS NOT HE WHO DOES NOT FEEL AFRAID, BUT HE WHO CONQUERS THAT FEAR.

NELSON MANDELA

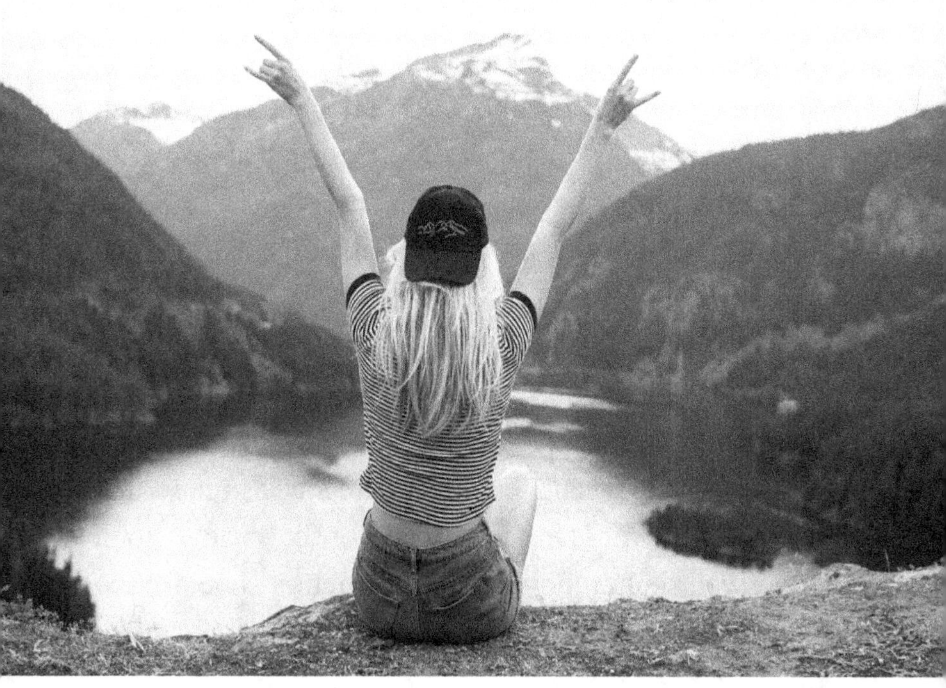

LIBERATING YOURSELF FROM EMOTIONAL EATING

Looking back at my emotional eating years, it is obvious how much I had struggled with food, how much of my life had revolved around food, and how all of that was entirely unnecessary.

The thing was, while I was living in a bubble, I thought this spectrum of emotions with respect to food was normal. Just like how some alcoholics or drug addicts see their addictions as under their control, I couldn't see the problem since I was living it. It was after resolving my food issues that I realized it really wasn't normal at all. That there *is* a better way, a more conscious path, one that doesn't involve food nor eating.

Just because others have the same problem doesn't mean there isn't a problem. It doesn't mean it's okay either. It just means that others are stuck in the same situation as you. Don't let norms of the society cloud over your better judgment. The solution shouldn't be to live in the problem, but to resolve it consciously.

Emotional eating doesn't have to persist. Just like me, you *can* break free from the chains binding you and food.

Here are the 21 tips that helped me build a healthy relationship with food and to live a life with confidence and inner courage.

42 | TIP #1 AWARENESS IS KEY

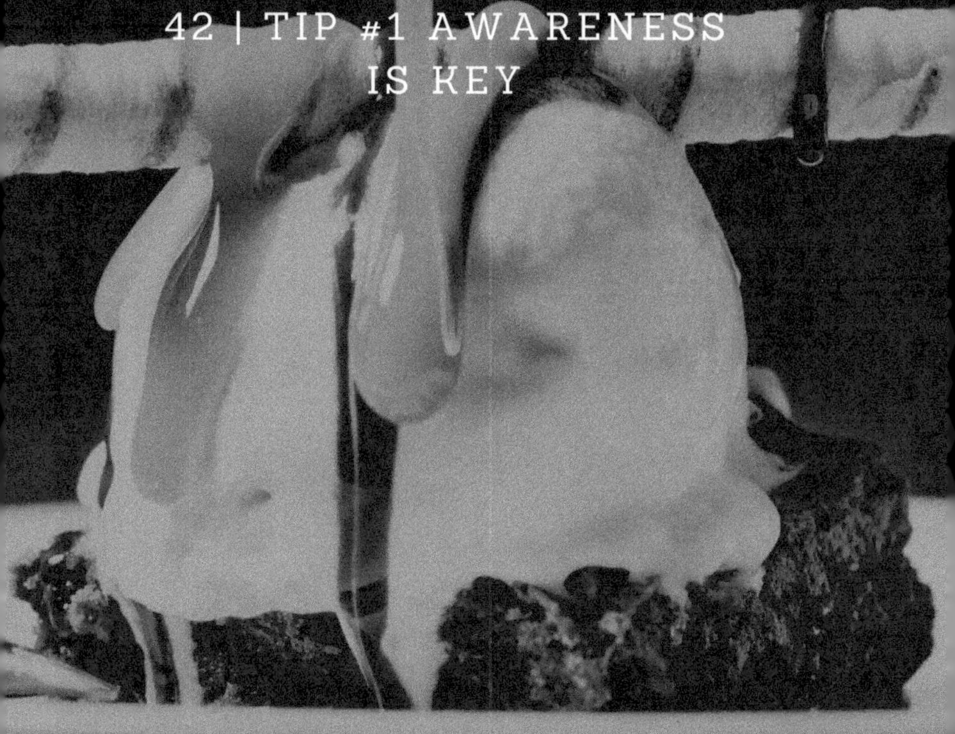

66

WHEN WE GET TOO CAUGHT UP IN THE BUSYNESS OF THE WORLD, WE LOSE CONNECTION WITH ONE ANOTHER – AND OURSELVES.

JACK KORNFIELD

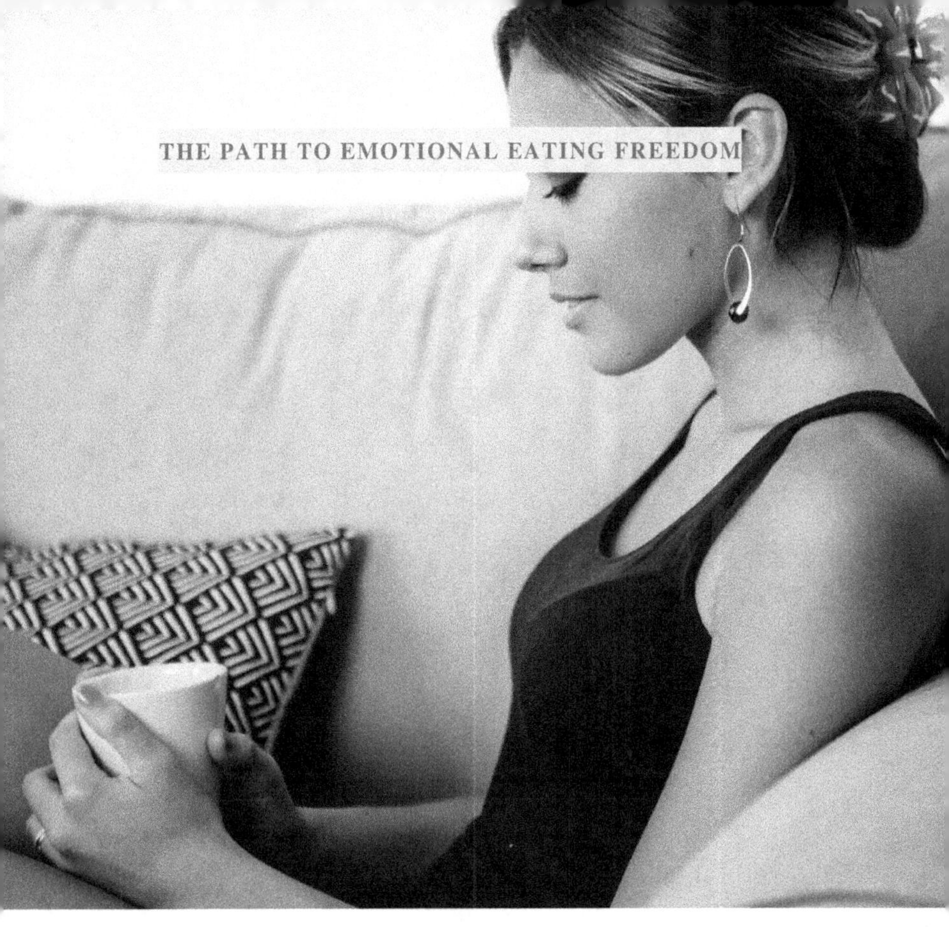

AWARENESS IS KEY

Awareness can be the most powerful aspect of change. Becoming more aware of how emotional eating plays out for you is the first step.

Emotional eating is sometimes called "mindless eating" because we often don't think about what we're doing and let our unconscious habits or drives take over. A mindful approach to eating can be helpful, but before you can put it into practice, you should become aware of how you feel right before you eat. The trick is to be more aware of why you're eating when you eat.

 **Solution**

One way to check in with yourself is to pause for a minute, step away from the kitchen or from being in close vicinity with any food, and simply breathe in and out slowly (mindful breathing) for 2 minutes.

The most basic way to do mindful breathing is simply to focus your attention on your breath. Focus on each inhale and exhale that you make. Count to 4 as you inhale then again count to 4 as you exhale.

You can do this while standing, but ideally you'll be sitting or even lying in a comfortable position. Just notice that this is happening and gently bring your attention back to your breath.

With your attention present in the moment, notice how your body feels. Ask yourself:
- Are you really hungry?
- Are you feeling stressed from your day?
- Are you tired?
- Are you bored?

- Is there something you ought to get done but dreading to do?
- Is it truly better to ignore a problem than deal with it repeatedly again in the future? Or, to solve it once and for all with courage, put it behind you and move forward in life feeling strong and happy with no negative baggage weighing you down?

There is no one around to judge you. Whatever the answer is, it is only for you to know so be honest with yourself.

If you realize you're eating for the wrong reasons, you can then move onto another approach to deal with your feelings.

Once you break the habit of mindlessly reaching for food, it becomes easier to put the next list of techniques into place.

47 | TIP #2 OVERCOME PROCRASTINATION

"

IN A MOMENT OF DECISION, THE BEST THING YOU CAN DO IS THE RIGHT THING TO DO, THE NEXT BEST THING IS THE WRONG THING, AND THE WORST THING YOU CAN DO IS NOTHING.

THEODORE ROOSEVELT

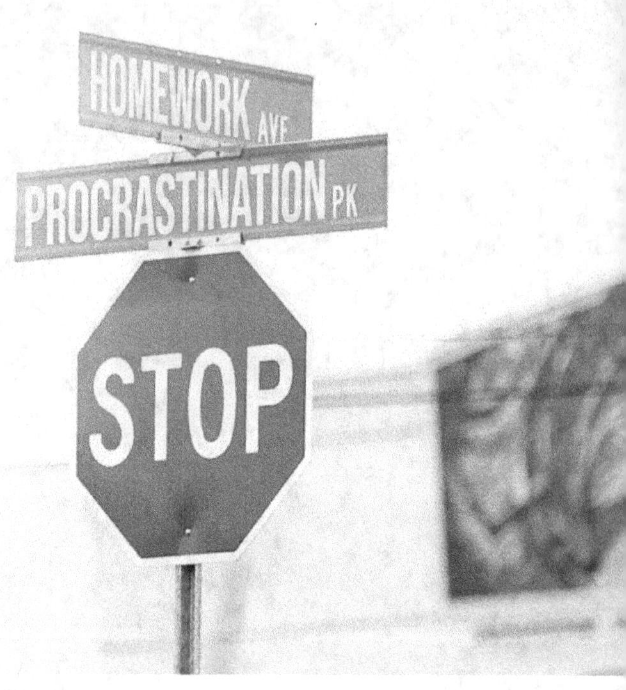

NOT NOW... MAYBE LATER?

We all delay the actions and choices we face. But for some of us, procrastination is our default setting. Far more than feeling overwhelmed and choosing to put something off, procrastination is a maladaptive lifestyle choice. It is our way of avoiding something and has the potential to lead to other problems in our lives, including overeating.

A hallmark of procrastination is seeking out distractions. We know we're avoiding a task so it helps to have an "excuse." You tell yourself you'll get to that something after you finish doing this other thing.

Oftentimes, when we're facing a deadline, there's kind of an unpleasant anxiety that comes with that. The anxiety is good because it helps us get things done, but the brain often looks for a short-term fix for anxiety, and certainly pleasurable food — which is often what snacks are, a sugary, salty, fatty tastiness — a very pleasurable signal for the brain.

As procrastination becomes more and more pervasive and thus dysfunctional, eating as a distraction transitions into overeating — and a dangerous cycle is created.

But there are psychiatrists who say the instinct to take a snack break can actually be a good one — if you choose your food wisely. They believe that it does serve a purpose.

When we want to increase cognitive capacity and mood, there are only a few ways to do that, and one of them is by eating simple carbs and sugar — there's an immediate boost in cognition that happens. Mood and focus go up, at least in the very short term.

 **1st Solution**

To make the most of your snack, psychiatrists recommend avoiding empty calories and instead munching on dark chocolate, a handful of nuts, an apple, or sipping green or herbal teas. Instead of having procrastinating hijack you, you are now using that desire as an opportunity to **enhance brain function.**

It is recommended to keep a range of healthy snacking options in your desk, which lets you get the benefits of a quick snack without losing momentum. Snacking often leads to chatting and then 30 minutes go by before you know it. Isn't it better if you spend 10 to 15 minutes focusing on getting your brain back in a way that enhances productivity and creativity so you can go on home and have a delicious dinner?

If you really want to stop procrastinating, it is also important to admit to yourself you have a problem. ("*I'm Trish, and I'm a procrastinator.*") Then, create a schedule — including snack breaks! — and stick to it, avoiding grazing in between.

It might be a little challenging at first, but you certainly can unlearn this behavior. Bear in mind, it gets easier after a week or so, and then it's a habit by the end of three to four weeks.

 **2nd Solution**

Use the 5 Second Rule by Mel Robbins.

The 5 Second Rule is simple. If you have an instinct to act on a goal, you **must physically move within 5 seconds or your brain will kill it**.

Let's say you wish to start waking up at 5am to get a jump start on your day (I wake up at 4am at times but I will admit that waking up that early doesn't get any easier). But as soon as I feel the vibration on my alarm and start to become somewhat functional, I immediately remember the rule. 5,4,3,2,1… and then I just go! It's not easy, but when I get to 1, I give myself no other option. Get up and get moving. I know the more time that passes, the more probable it is that I hit the snooze button and fall back asleep. And that is the last thing that I want.

Whatever task or project that you know you need to get done but find yourself dragging your feet to get a jump start on things, try the 5 Second Rule.

Will you ever really feel like doing whatever that it is you don't feel like doing?

Probably not.

Why?

Because if it was so easy and pleasurable in the first place, you would have done it a long time ago without overthinking it.

What's the benefit of using the 5 Second Rule?

As you start to get things moving along and start seeing results, chances are, you will be more inclined to do *more* because now you know (and see for yourself) that by putting procrastination behind you and take immediate massive action (regardless how mundane the task may seem), things get **done**.

54 | TIP #3 KNOW YOUR CALORIES

> **DO THE BEST YOU CAN UNTIL YOU KNOW BETTER. THEN WHEN YOU KNOW BETTER, DO BETTER.**

MAYA ANGELOU

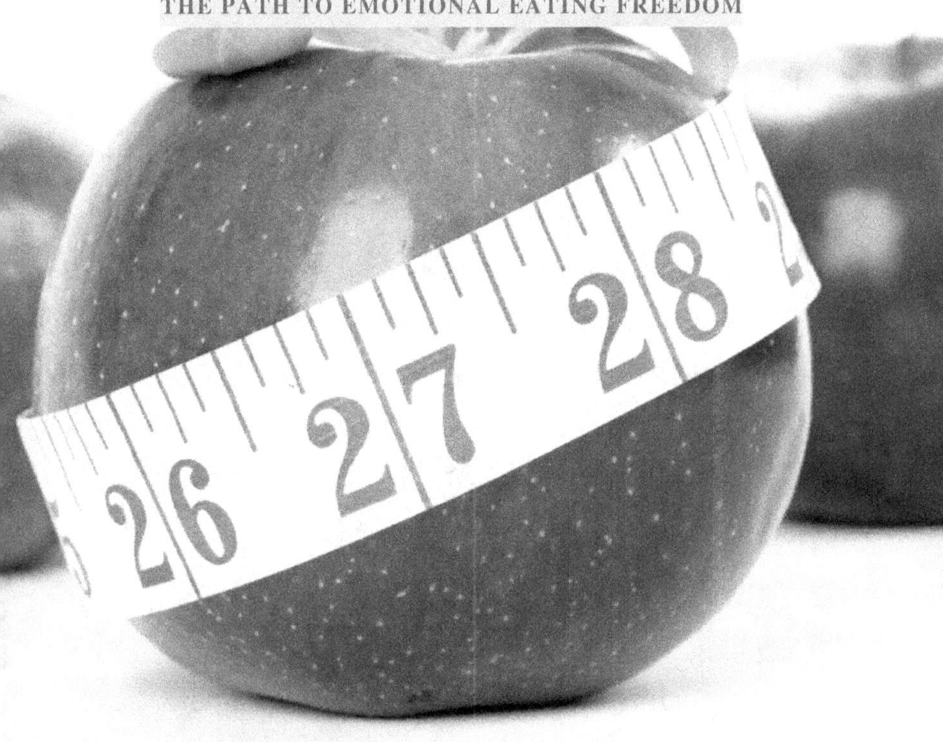

IMPORTANCE OF UNDERSTANDING CALORIES

What is a calorie and why is it important to know how many calories there are in certain foods?

A calorie is actually a unit of heat energy. That's right. We think of calories as just things that are in food and all foods have calories. But your body sees calories as energy and it's energy to produce heat.

Heat energy is what really fuels our body just the same way that gasoline is what fuels your car's energy.

All foods have calories and different foods have different amounts of calories. Calories are provided by fat, carbohydrate, and protein.

Fats have the highest concentration of calories. That's nine calories per gram of pure fat. **Protein** and **carbohydrates** each have four calories per gram of pure protein or pure carbohydrate. **Alcohol**, pure alcohol, has seven calories per gram. So understanding the role of calories in your diet can help you balance the amount of calories you consume against the amount of calories you burn, thus helping you achieve your weight management goals.

You can find out the calories in foods by looking at the calorie label or the nutrition facts panel on packages of processed foods. They will all have the number of calories per serving and the portion size per serving. By using these information provided, you can help educate yourself on the estimated amount of calories you're taking in per day and help you maintain or achieve your weight loss goals.

But how do you know whether you are eating just the right amount of calories, undereating or overeating?

 ### Solution

Get a calorie counting app and start logging down your meals and drinks in a day. There are tons of free and paid apps out there to choose from.

If you prefer using a journal, that's also fine.

Based on your ideal healthy body mass index (BMI) and daily activity level, you can determine the estimated calories you should be taking in.

WARNING!

In no way am I encouraging anyone to become obsessed with calorie counting and suck the joy out of eating. Though it pains me to say this, but I was once in that exact dark hole, obsessively counting calories, fearful of eating even one extra calorie than the recommended amount of calories suggested for me (based on my BMI) to maintain my ideal weight. I can safely say it isn't a very nice place to be. Therefore, I definitely **DO NOT** wish that for you.

The point of noting down what you eat and drink is to be more *mindful* of what you are consuming in a day. Knowing what you are eating and being aware of its nutritional value is part of the concept of eating mindfully and making smart choices for your health. Having a rough overview of what you eat and drink through a food journal or calorie counting app is better than having no idea at all.

Many people underestimate how many calories are hidden in many processed foods and soft drinks. A small piece of chocolate here, a sweet there, 1 glass of soft drink, a glass of wine there, and it all adds up.

It is simple maths. Your body can only use up so much of the energy you feed it with. Any excess is either excreted through bowel movement or stored as unhealthy fats.

To maintain a healthy weight, you need to consume about the same amount of energy as you would exert in a day.

To reduce weight, you need to consume slightly lesser to create a deficit. (Warning! Again, don't go overboard and become underweight. That is **not** what

I am trying to encourage any one to do. The purpose of knowing your calories is purely to be more mindful of what you are consuming in a day and to know better whether what you are consuming is serving or harming your body.)

Your body is not a thing for you to abuse, it is a tool blessed upon you to give you the opportunity to experience life.

Treat it well by nourishing it and it will serve you well in return in the long run.

EMPTY CALORIES

Ever heard of foods containing "empty calories"? If not, then now is the time to empower yourself with this knowledge to have a better understanding about calories and the way it functions in our bodies.

It is very important to know that **not all calories are equal**.

Many of the packaged foods you'll find at the grocery store contain empty calories. This means they have little nutritional value. Instead, they give your body mostly solid fats and added sugars, which can lead to weight gain and nutritional deficiencies.

Not only that, the excess sugar, especially in beverages, will *not* fill you up or make you less hungry (it will only fill you up for a *very* short time!), but it will add significantly to your daily calorie intake. The saturated fat isn't healthy for your body and won't provide you with the healthy fats your body needs, but it will pack a hefty dose of calories into your diet!

Some **good examples of empty calories** are:
- Soft drinks, sports drinks, and other sweetened drinks
- Fried foods
- Cookies, cake, donuts, and similar desserts
- Processed and fatty meats like sausages, hot dogs, and bacon
- Cream and high-fat dairy products, like cheese and whole milk

Let's be real though, everyone (me included) eats empty calories now and then. You can have that occasional treat at a special event or as a small serving from time to time. The **key** is to limit your intake of empty calories, and fill your diet with lower sugar, lower fat foods that give your body the nutrients it needs.

Some **great examples of fresh, wholesome foods** are:

- Fresh fruits without added sugars
- Low-calorie salad dressing on a fresh vegetable salad (without cheese)
- Lean, skinless chicken and turkey (not fried)
- Substituting olive oil instead of butter
- Baked potato instead of fries or chips
- A slice of whole grain bread, instead of a croissant or muffin

Many of these foods will help you to feel full longer, so you'll be less tempted to reach for the empty calorie foods. Try to omit those sources of empty calories as much as you can, and you may start to see more results from your weight loss plan. It's a great habit to adopt as you strive for a healthier weight and lifestyle.

Eating healthy doesn't mean it has to be bland or tasteless. Try to be creative with food. Experiment with your meals by adding a dash of low fat sauce, pepper, spices, and a variety of herbs to make your meals more pleasurable.

Now it's time to put on your thinking cap.

What are your favourite fresh foods? What other healthy wholesome food can you think of to make your meals both healthy and bursting with flavour?

Challenge yourself to list out at least 10 more.

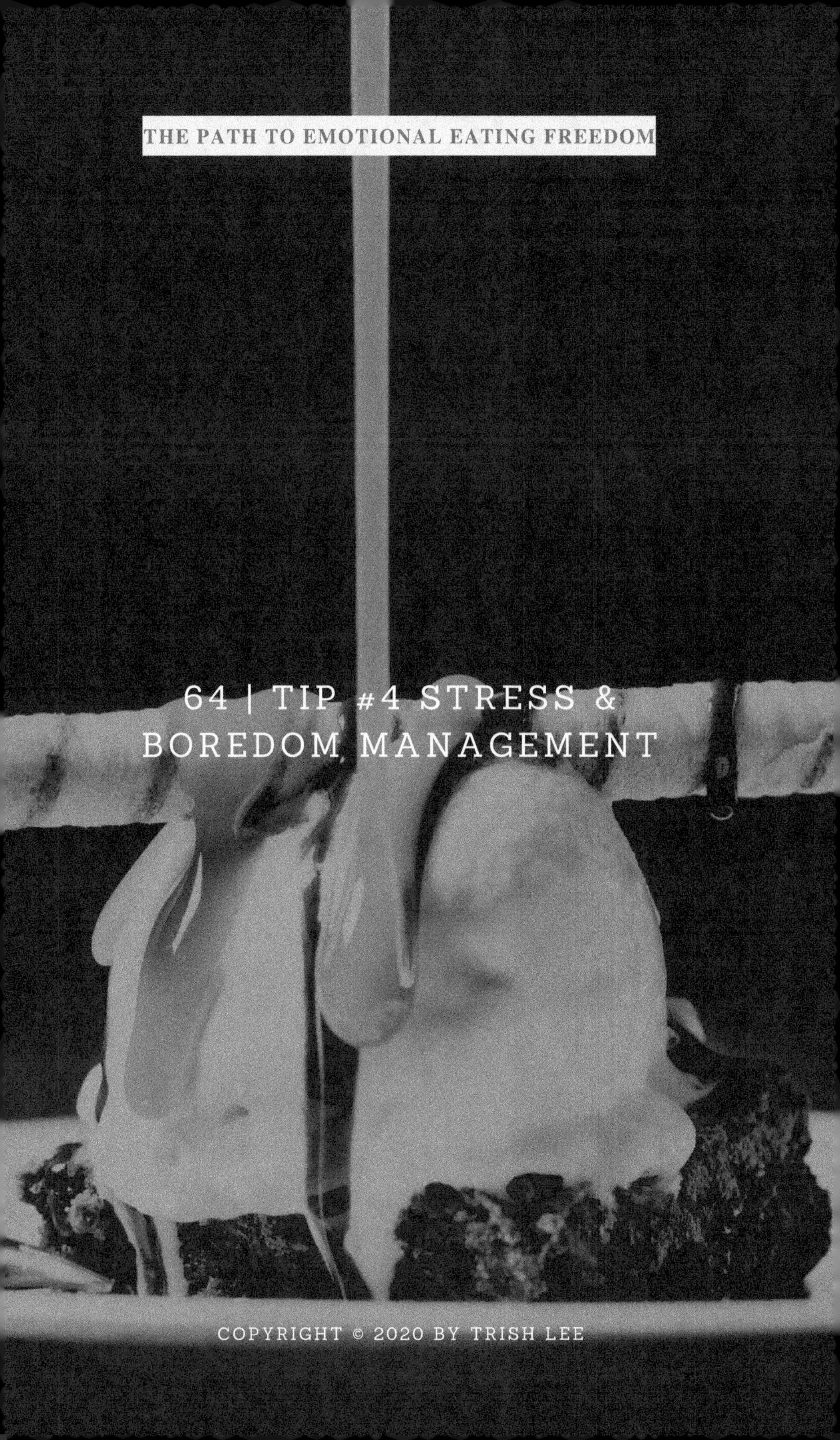

64 | TIP #4 STRESS & BOREDOM MANAGEMENT

"

STRESS IS CAUSED BY BEING 'HERE' BUT WANTING TO BE 'THERE'.

ECKHART TOLLE

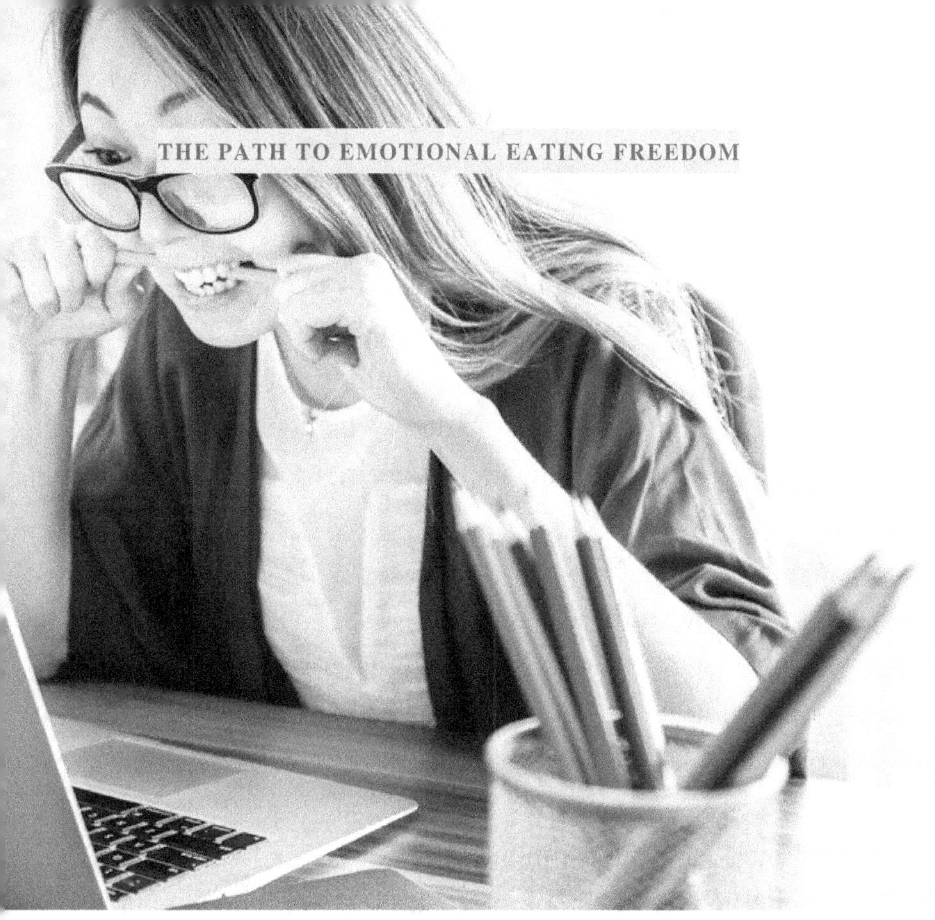

CREATE YOUR LIST OF OTHER OPTIONS

My best tool to combat stress eating or eating out of pure boredom is to create a list of other activities that will make us feel better without the guilt that overeating often brings.

Research tells us that there are other things that will

create a response similar to the one junk food brings without the guilt and frustration of overeating. These are things like connection, mindfulness, meditation, exercise, and (if you're really going for it) romance. These things will also naturally dampen your threat response system and help you manage stress more effectively.

 **Solution**

For a start, make a list of activities you might enjoy that don't involve preparing, eating or shopping for food.

One of the simplest, easiest and healthiest alternatives to emotional eating is walking: regular walking, speed walking, walking on a treadmill, walking your dog. Craft activities like knitting or felting not only pass the time and give you something physical to do, but allow you to be creative and productive.

Some other suggestions for you to consider are:

- Crossword puzzles
- Games (eg: Chess, cards, games on your phone, etc)

- Turn on your favourite music and just dance your heart out!
- Swim
- Yoga
- Journalling
- Soak in a bathtub
- Manicure or pedicure
- Get a massage
- Flip through your collection of photos and videos that make you smile
- Watch a sitcom
- Read a book
- Draw or paint
- Learn a new language or skill (through YouTube or by signing up for a program online)
- Visit the zoo
- Connect with someone you've lost touch with
- Call a friend or family
- Gardening
- Colour an adult colouring book
- Create your bucket list (then start ticking things off one at a time!)

Can you think of any other fun or meaningful activities to add to this list?

Don't be afraid to add them to the list and make it your own.

Hang this list in prominent places around your office, home, your car or save it as a note in your phone to remind you of all the activities that you can do to release stress or overcome boredom without the need to use food as a form of comfort.

Gentle reminder: After you feel your stress reduce, do make it a *must* to manage the problem that lead you to want to binge eat mindlessly in the first place. It must not be immediately, but make time and take the effort to settle it once and for all so that it won't keep reappearing in your life and sway you away from your efforts of living a healthier lifestyle.

70 | TIP #5 SELF-COMPASSION

WE CAN'T HATE OURSELVES INTO A VERSION OF OURSELVES WE CAN LOVE.

LORI DESCHENE

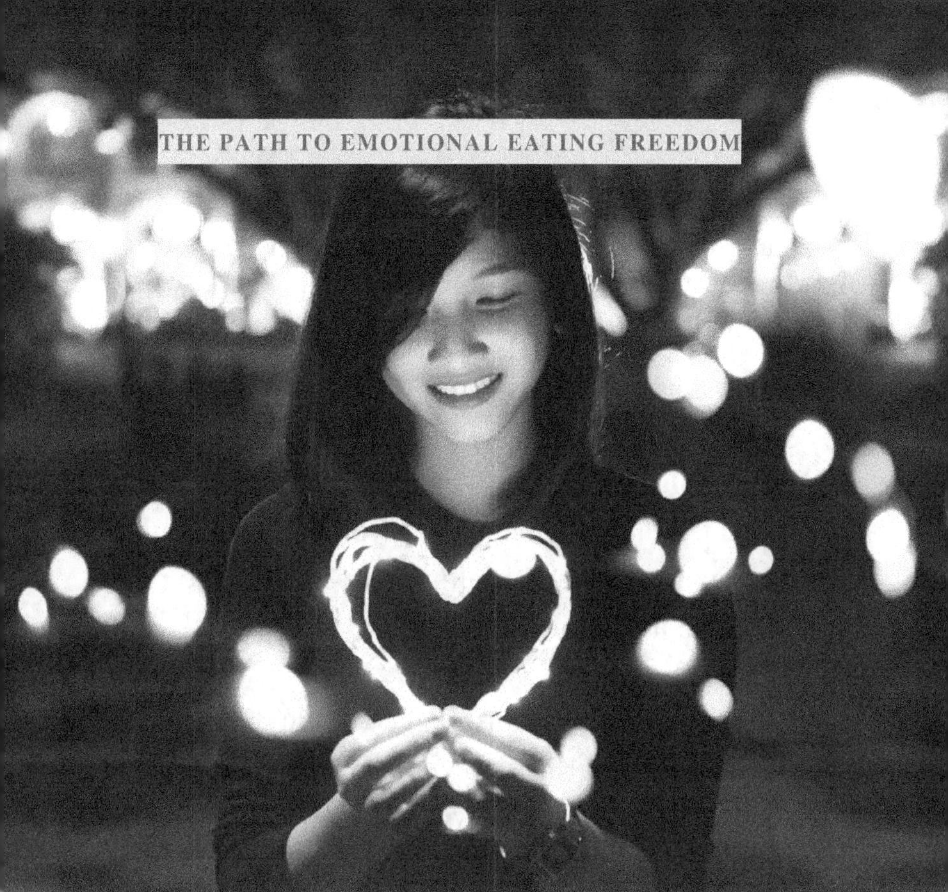

LOVE YOUR WAY TO HAPPINESS

Moving from self-loathing to self-love can seem an impossible task when binge eating has a grip on your life.

For many people, especially women, binge eating can seem stronger than the power to control it. Feelings of being held captive by helplessness to make changes or to stay disciplined in their weight management plan can lead to frustration, hopelessness, anxiety, emptiness, self-hatred, and depression.

 ## Solution

If you tend to tell yourself that you will love yourself when you are fit and healthy, then it is time to pause and think about this statement.

By continuously "punishing" yourself because you think you'll never be good enough or you'll never hit your ideal weight, how will you ever become the fit and healthy person that you want to be?

For a change, try loving yourself and see what beautiful changes can happen.

Love yourself enough to know that the **choices you make today, will determine your tomorrow**.

Love yourself enough to trust that good things take time, that through little positive changes in your eating habits everyday, it will pay off in good time.

Love yourself enough to forgive yourself if you do indulge a little sometimes, that it is not the end of the world. What is more important, is to have the courage to get back on track and come back stronger every time.

75 | TIP #6 THE NOW OR NEVER MENTALITY

THERE IS A FINE LINE BETWEEN LOVING LIFE AND BEING GREEDY FOR IT.

MAYA ANGELOU

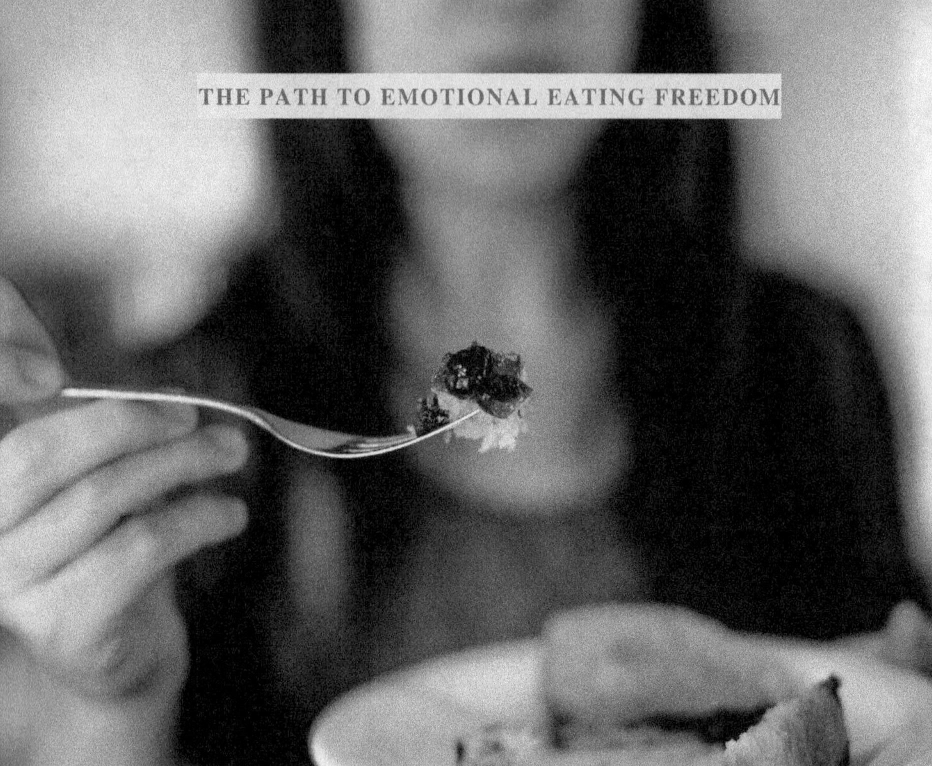

BUT WHAT IF I NEVER GET TO EAT IT AGAIN?

Ever went to a nice restaurant, ate something nice, then thought, "Hey that's delicious! Maybe I should have more of that because who knows when I'm gonna have it again?"

If you have, you aren't alone. Even I am guilty of having these types of thoughts at times.

The food tastes *sooooo* good that even if the portion may be too big, you force yourself to finish it. Or worse still, you feel it tasted out of this world, thus you ordered a second portion despite the fact you're already full to the brim.

While it is not wrong to have a *little* more of something that we rarely get to indulge in, people who love food or have binge eating tendencies will find that this type of thinking often makes them overeat unknowingly.

 **Solution**

If you find yourself having these thoughts the next time, ask yourself this, can you eat your whole life time's meals in ONE sitting just because you are scared you won't have enough food or get to eat the same delicious food in the future?

Obviously, no.

We aren't camels. Our bodies are not built to store food and go without eating for 6 or 7 months.

The best way to deal with the urge to indulge in food that you really like again, is by either:

- **Packing** the food to take home (you can enjoy it the next day), or
- **Plan** it in your journal or appointment calendar to visit the restaurant again the next week or month to enjoy the meal again.

If you are on holiday in a foreign country and find yourself battling with this same dilemma, obviously it can prove to be a little more tricky because packing the food or planning to have it again soon may not be possible.

By asking myself the following questions, it has helped me to gain more control over my cravings:

By stuffing my face now, will I get upset and disappointed with myself for putting on an extra 5kgs by the time I get home?

Do I really want to end my holiday on a sour note?

Is it really true that I will never be able to enjoy this food again? Truth is, no. Most countries have restaurants offering cuisines from all over the world.

In any case, if the food is connected to a specific

location and emotion (eg: a place where your partner asked you for your hand in marriage), and the only way to relive that moment is by eating that exact same food in that exact same spot, then make it a goal to budget for another trip to this holiday destination in the near future.

"If it is important to you, you will find a way. If not, you'll find an excuse."
- Ryan Blair

All this said, you can see now that there really is no reason to allow this "now or never" mentality to make you overeat anymore.

81 | TIP #7 GIVING UP WHEN WEIGHT LOSS PLATEAUS

THERE IS NO FAILURE EXCEPT IN NO LONGER TRYING.

ELBERT HUBBARD

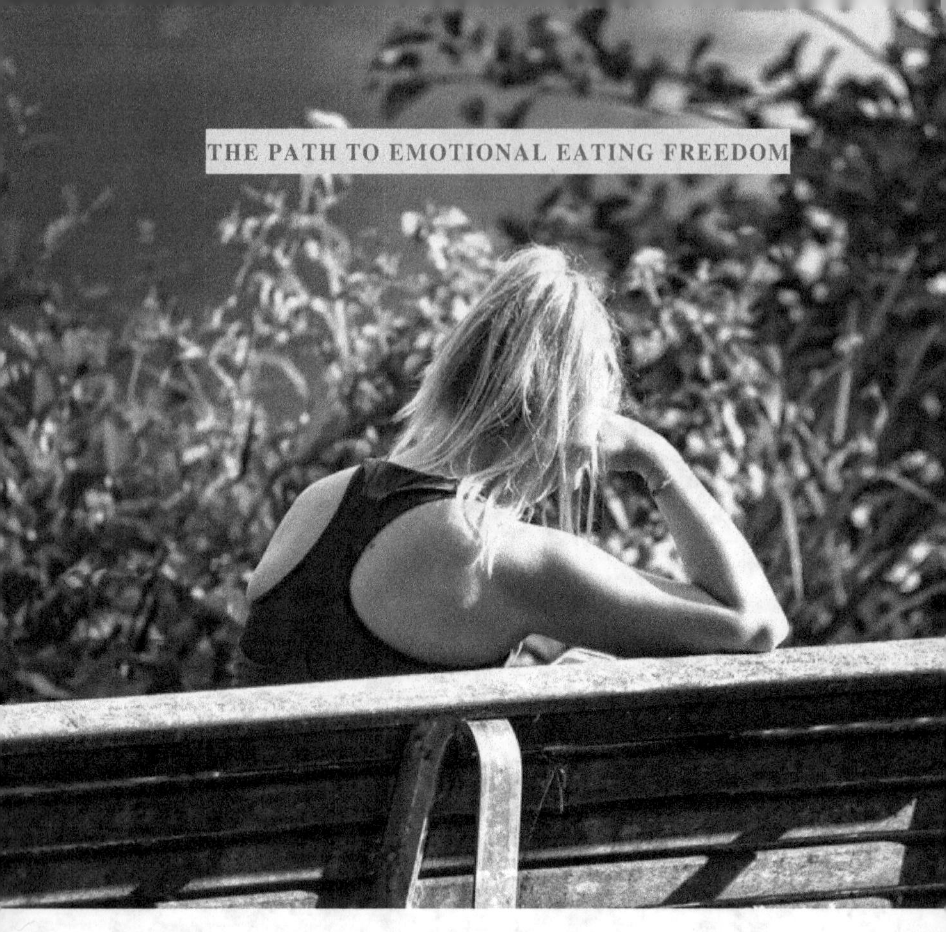

WHY EVEN BOTHER TRYING?

Just because you've tried once or twice or maybe because you aren't seeing results as fast as your friends in the quest to achieve your target weight doesn't mean that it can't be done.

As tempting as it can be to drown your sorrows in food, remind yourself that doing so will only make you undo all the progress (however small it may be) you have achieved.

If you feel the urge to starve yourself to punish yourself for hitting a plateau, understand that doing so will only cause you to have a strong urge to binge eat like crazy later on.

Rather than starve yourself or condemn yourself, remind yourself that it is **perfectly normal** for our body weights to fluctuate from one day to another.

Research has shown that a five-pound weight shift is typical for most people day-to-day, but that the number on the scale can change by as much as 20 pounds depending on your body size. So why the big swing? And what causes these frustrating weight fluctuations from day to day?

Here are the factors that contribute to an increase or decrease on the scale:

- Weight fluctuation from **sodium** (High salt foods can cause water retention)
- Weight fluctuation from **carbohydrates** (For every gram of carbohydrate you consume, your body retains about three grams of water in order to store the fuel source)

- Weight fluctuation from **food weight** (According to some experts, consuming two cups of water—from beverages or water in food—increases your weight by one pound)
- Weight fluctuation from **bowel movements** (Though not very significant, it still plays a minor role in weight fluctuation)
- Weight fluctuation from **exercise** (If you notice that you lose weight consistently after exercise, you may want to come up with an improved hydration plan. Why? Because fluids lost during exercise should be replaced.
- Weight fluctuation from **medication** (Certain medications may cause you to gain weight. If this occurs, don't stop taking the medication. Instead, talk to your doctor or pharmacist)
- Weight fluctuation from your **menstrual cycle** (Studies have linked fluctuations in estradiol and progesterone (your ovarian hormones) to changes in binge eating and emotional eating)
- Weight fluctuation from **alcohol** intake (Researchers have found that alcohol can cause your body to retain fluids from food and drinks that you consume)

 **1st Solution**

One tip that has helped me come to terms with the

fluctuation in my weight is by having a healthy weight range in mind, rather than having only a very *specific* number.

For example, I am fine if my weight fluctuates between 123 - 130lb. The range is reasonable enough for me to eat healthy and not feel like I am off track from maintaining my ideal weight. I don't penalize myself to have say 125lb as my target goal and it is only that number I need to maintain or not at all.

Another important point to keep in mind if you are exercising or doing heavy house chores regularly is that both muscle and fat increases your mass, so your weight gain isn't necessarily always bad.

To be successful, you have to believe in yourself and stay motivated by an ongoing belief that you can accomplish anything you set out to do. You can't be happy and successful all the time; that's not realistic. But you can learn to focus on your successes, not on your failures. You can push yourself to keep seeking solutions rather than losing hope or giving up when you hit an obstacle.

Other people can help to a large degree, but it's up to

you to find your strengths and use them to do the inner work, the emotional work that only you can do.

2nd Solution

The power of visualization

Visualization techniques have been used by successful people to visualize their desired outcomes for ages.

The practice has even given some high achievers what seems like super-powers, helping them create their dream lives by accomplishing one goal or task at a time with hyper focus and complete confidence.

In fact, we all have this awesome power, but most of us have never been taught to use it effectively. Elite athletes use it. The super-rich use it. And peak performers in all fields now use it. That power is called **visualization**.

The daily practice of visualizing your dreams as already complete can rapidly accelerate your achievement of those dreams, goals, and ambitions. Using visualization techniques to focus on your goals and desires yields 4 very important benefits.

1.) It **activates your creative subconscious** which will start generating creative ideas to achieve your goal.

2.) It **programs your brain** to more readily perceive and recognize the resources you will need to achieve your dreams.

3.) It **activates the law of attraction**, thereby drawing into your life the people, resources, and circumstances you will need to achieve your goals.

4.) It **builds your internal motivation** to take the necessary actions to achieve your dreams.

Visualization is really quite simple. You sit in a comfortable position, close your eyes and imagine — in as vivid detail as you can — what you would be looking at if the dream you have were already realized. Imagine being inside of yourself, looking out through your eyes at the ideal result.

Whenever I hit a weight loss plateau, I visualized the healthy weight that I want to achieve.

Back when I was a teenager, the celebrity who

inspired me was actress, author, entrepreneur, and philanthropist Jessica Alba. I used to visualize myself as having her height, weight, and looks. Just my personal thoughts, I felt her weight was very proportionate to her height, her facial features gorgeous, and her personality super likeable.

Using the power of visualization has helped me to overcome moments of feeling "stuck" or in times when I feel like my efforts were not fruitful.

It gave me new hope and new motivation to **keep going and keep trying.**

If you find visualizing a person as your desired role model too challenging, another powerful visualization technique is to create a photograph or picture of yourself with your goal, as if it were already completed, and have that photo placed at prominent areas in your house or office to further motivate you towards achieving your greatness.

If say one of your goals is to own a new car, take your camera down to your local auto dealer and have a picture taken of yourself sitting behind the wheel of your dream car. If your goal is to visit Paris, find a picture or poster of the Eiffel Tower and cut out a photo of yourself and place it onto the picture.

What is the ideal weight that you'd like to achieve? Does any particular celebrity or friend come to mind who you look up to as a role model for your ideal weight?

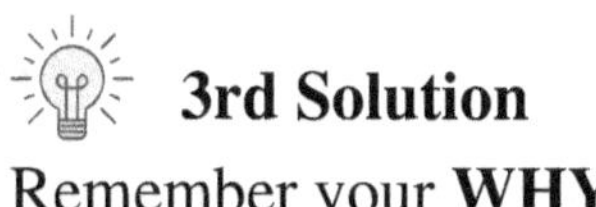 **3rd Solution**

Remember your **WHY**

In times when you feel like giving up on building a healthier relationship with food or maybe to achieve your desired weight, remind yourself **why** you even started on this journey in the first place.

It shouldn't be a small, insignificant "why", it should be a **BIG** "why". A reason that *really* matters to you.

For me, I know my WHYs as clear as day. These are the reasons why I could achieve my goal weight when I was a teenager and why I could lose over 26 pounds within a year after giving birth.

   1. I want to **feel strong** and never let anyone have the chance to use physical force on me ever again

2. I want to **feel energized** throughout my day

3. I want to **look good for myself** because that is what gives me confidence to feel like a million bucks

It's time to dig deep and write out your "why". Why do you want to stop emotional eating? Why does it matter to you so much?

92 | TIP #8 THE IMPORTANCE OF SLEEP

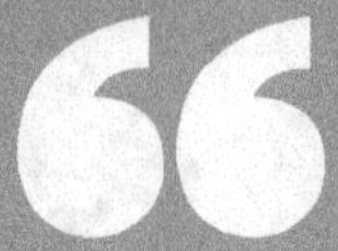

SLEEP IS THAT GOLDEN CHAIN THAT TIES HEALTH AND OUR BODIES TOGETHER.

THOMAS DEKKER

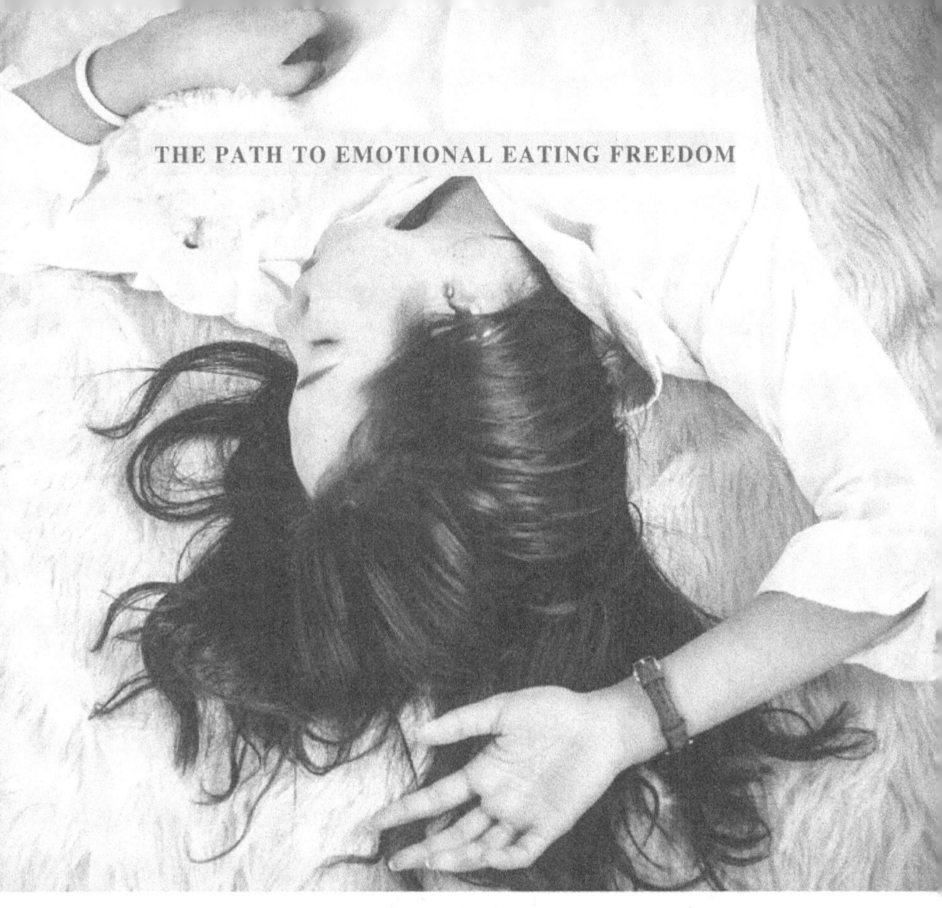

YOU SNOOZE, YOU WIN

Not getting enough sleep doesn't just make you tired. It also makes you fat, according to scientists.

The three key impacts that studies have gathered from lack of sleep are:
- People who only got five hours sleep a night gained two pounds in a week
- When sleep is deprived, people eat less breakfast but more snacks

          94

- Lack of sleep slows the metabolism, causing the body to burn fewer calories

 **Solutions**

1) Consider if your sleep struggles more on the side of **quantity** (getting enough hours) or **quality** (how well you sleep)

Even modest improvements in either dimension can make a difference. Sleep quantity problems often require different solutions than quality problems. For example, sleep quantity might be improved by changes that help you fall asleep more quickly (e.g., relaxing or meditating before bedtime or taking your sedating medicines at night). Alternatively, sleep quality may be improved by reducing nighttime light exposure and addressing anything that might be causing you to wake up at night (e.g., minimize fluids in the evening).

2) "**Tap into your inner child**" for better sleep

This means thinking back to the time of your life when you slept the best and recreating those circumstances as closely as possible in the present. Children often sleep better than adults, for example, because they have more consistent sleep schedules, routines their parents practice with them before bed, and relaxation strategies parents use to help children fall asleep (e.g., reading them bedtime stories). In a present-day form, we may benefit from the childhood strategies that worked for us in the past.

3) **Change your attitude and emotions** about sleep

In a competitive culture like ours, sleep is often treated as a waste of time or an obstacle to productivity. Compare that attitude to a person who sees sleep as the precious time during which they learn, heal, and grow – all indisputably supported by research – and guess which attitude contributes more to sleep problems.

4) The Power of a **20-Minute Nap**

Also known as a "power nap", something I highly recommend people who work long hours and especially parents who don't have the luxury of getting 8 hours uninterrupted sleep at night to apply.

Researchers and nap-takers tout those 20 minutes of

rest as the holy grail of nap length.

Why?

Sleep experts suggest after 30 minutes, the body can fall into a deeper sleep, even risking feeling more tired than how you previously were.

And while 20 minutes may seem like a meek window of shuteye, power naps have shown to:
- combat against fatigue
- promote a greater physical and mental well-being
- increase emotional functioning
- improve mood and heighten concentration levels
- develop adequate sleeping patterns at bedtime
- strengthen interpersonal relationships
- lessen the risk of weight gain

When you feel more energized and focused, you're able to make more mindful decisions where your health is concerned, thus curbing the urge to binge eat mindlessly.

98 | TIP #9 REWARD THYSELF

"

I AM NOT A PRODUCT OF MY CIRCUMSTANCE. I AM A PRODUCT OF MY DECISIONS.

STEPHEN COVEY

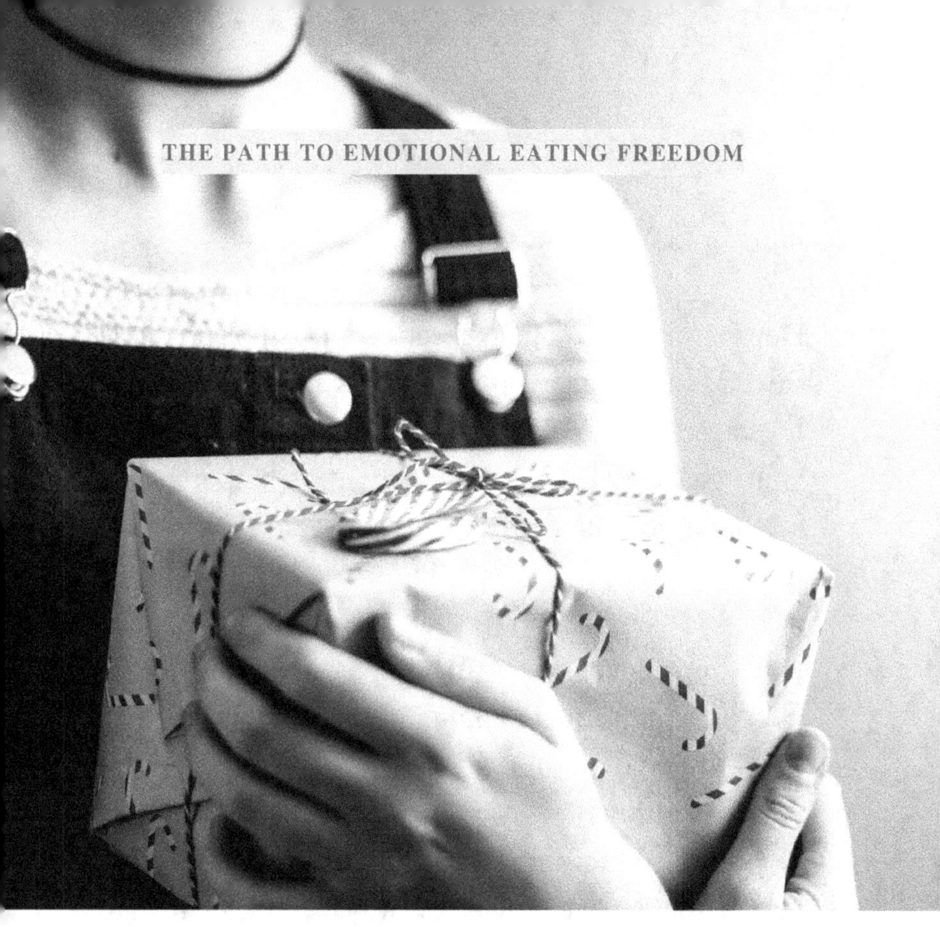

WHY GIFT YOURSELF SOMETHING YOU'LL HATE YOURSELF FOR?

For most of us, our parents probably used to reward us with food whenever we got good grades or when we did something right.

While that sounds nice, it can also cause us to associate eating as the only way to reward ourselves in order to feel good.

Don't get me wrong, the carrot and stick principle (reward and punish system) still works and you can leverage it to build good habits that help you reach your goals faster. This is why it is important to celebrate your hard work and to reward yourself for the effort that you have put in.

However, there are many other ways to reward yourself apart from indulging in food and wine.

 **Solutions**

No matter how small a milestone you may have achieved, here are a list of ways you can reward yourself for a job well done to motivate yourself to go further:

- Try something new that you've always wanted to try
- Do a fun activity with your kids
- Go to a carnival, festival, or arts and crafts show
- Go for a concert
- Plan for your next staycation or holiday overseas
- Go to an art gallery

- Indulge your senses with a season pass to the theater or opera
- Go to a park you've never been to before
- Marathon your favorite show on Netflix
- Plan a night out with your friends
- Play pool
- Go on a boat ride
- Play your favorite online game
- Attend a drag show
- Go for a karaoke session
- Play bowling
- Attend a sporting event
- Take a pottery / jewelry making / knitting / photography class
- Buy yourself some fresh flowers
- Get yourself a pet
- Go shopping (but set a reasonable budget for yourself to avoid overspending)
- Plan your next staycation or holiday
- Do volunteer work or donate to a cause you support (this is an awesome way of passing on positive vibes onto others while attracting more good karma your way)

These are just some of the fun ways to reward yourself that has worked for me and my coaching clients.

What other creative ways comes to your mind? Write it down and work towards rewarding yourself with it the next time you hit another milestone. Good luck and have fun celebrating!

104 | TIP #10 THE "ULTIMATE" DIET PLAN

"

YOUR LIFE DOES NOT GET BETTER BY CHANCE, IT GETS BETTER BY CHANGE.

JIM ROHN

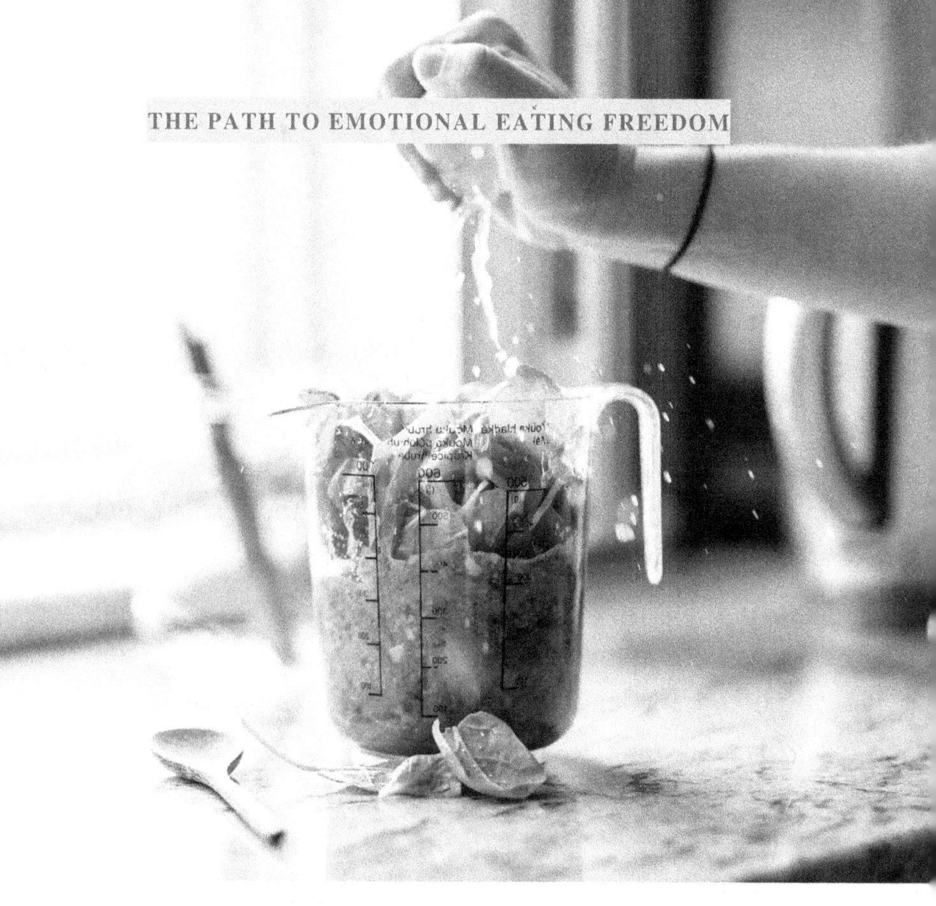

THE "RIGHT" DIET PLAN

Have you ever followed your doctor's weight loss nutrition plan to a T, only to stubbornly remain at the exact same weight -- or worse, gain weight?

And of course, thanks to social media, advertisements, influencers and the likes, trying to constantly sell us the idea that the Keto diet, Paleo diet, Vegan diet, Atkins diet, and what have you is *the* one and only best diet for you?

Well, apparently, that is not true at all.

New research says this kind of one-size-fits-all approach may not cut it. Different people, even identical twins (who have nearly the exact same DNA), may respond to the same foods very differently, the researchers found—complicating decades of weight loss and health advice, and potentially leaving consumers with more questions than answers.

Tim Spector, a professor of genetic epidemiology at King's College London says that recommendations, medically and public-health wise, have just been assuming that if people follow the standard plan, they'll lose weight and develop fewer chronic diseases. But in actual fact, that thinking has now been exposed as completely flawed.

The study's results were presented in mid 2019 at the American Society for Nutrition conference. Researchers tracked about 1,100 U.S. and U.K. adults, including 240 pairs of twins, for two weeks.

They monitored participants' blood sugar, insulin and fat levels after they ate pre-formulated meals like muffins and glucose drinks; tested the microbes living in their guts; and tracked their sleep and exercise.

Foods that spiked one person's blood sugar or kept their fat levels elevated for hours didn't necessarily do the same for the person dining next to them—even if they were twins. Individuals even had different responses to the same meals when they were eaten at different times of the day. These results suggest that nutrition facts alone cannot predict how a certain food will affect health and weight.

It doesn't mean you throw all nutrition advice out. There are some guidelines and recommendations around the world that many people agree on, including eating plenty of produce and fiber, and cutting back on calories and ultra-processed foods. But plenty of lingering nutrition questions—

- *Is it okay to skip breakfast?*
- *Does fasting work?*

- *Is a low-carb or low-fat diet better for weight loss?*

may not have one single answer.

Solution

Practice tuning in to your body's needs. Personally, I've tried countless of diet plans and most of them only ended up making me feel more hungry, more stressed up, and made me gain more weight.

Some nutritionists say you feel full after eating avocado, banana, and eggs. Frankly, it doesn't work for me at all. In fact the opposite happens and I end up overeating.

After much trial and error, these are the 2 basic eating principles that has helped me shed all my pregnancy weight as well as aided me in maintaining my ideal weight.

1) The 80/20 Diet

Essentially it means that 80% of the food you eat should be a healthy variety of vegetables, fruits, lean meats, and fish. The remaining 20% can be a little more indulgent, like a slice of pepperoni pizza or a couple of cocktails with friends at a bar. It's best to stick to foods you truly love. Those treats will give you the biggest boost of satisfaction

2) Semi fasting

I eat dinner by 5pm everyday then not another morsel until breakfast time at 6 or 7am the next day. I feel that by doing so, I wake up feeling fresh, light, and energised the next morning.

When I eat a late dinner (any time after 6pm), my stomach feels stuffed and uncomfortable.

I'm a breakfast person I admit. But interestingly enough, when my husband eats breakfast with me, he ends up feeling too full for the rest of the day. Like I said, all our bodies are just made differently. So what works for me, may not work for you, and vice versa.

The best thing you can do is, try different diets for 1-2 months to get a clearer idea if it works for you or not. It doesn't matter what diet plan it is (just please avoid any extreme diets that leaves you feeling starved or depressed), give it your best try and don't throw in the towel too early. Because if you do, you won't truly know if it works or not.

Another key point I want to emphasise here, is that just because a food is labelled as 'healthy', doesn't mean that you can eat it as much as you like and not have to worry about weight gain.

That thinking is false through and through.

I once had a client who asked me why her Keto diet was not working for her. She read that avocados contain healthy fats and so she has been eating a few of them everyday.

Here's the thing, even the healthiest of food contains calories. Just because a food is healthy, doesn't mean you eat more of it in extreme. Anything in extreme can and will cause either complications in your digestive system or weight gain.

Even vitamins, an overload of vitamins and minerals can hurt you. Too much vitamin C or zinc could cause nausea, diarrhea, and stomach cramps. Too much selenium could lead to hair loss, gastrointestinal upset, fatigue, and mild nerve damage.

Learn to eat everything in moderation. Again, sometimes there is just no one size fits all solution. If something isn't working for you, it doesn't mean there is something wrong with you. It just means that perhaps there is a different more effective diet for you.

Therefore, don't lose hope. If a diet plan didn't work for you, pick yourself up and try again until you find a diet plan or eating routine that suits your body's needs. Take time to tune in to your body's needs and respect what it is telling you or making you feel. This inner voice will guide you well.

113 | TIP #11 SLOW DOWN

"

EVERY DAY BRINGS A CHOICE: TO PRACTICE STRESS OR TO PRACTICE PEACE.

JOAN BORYSENKO

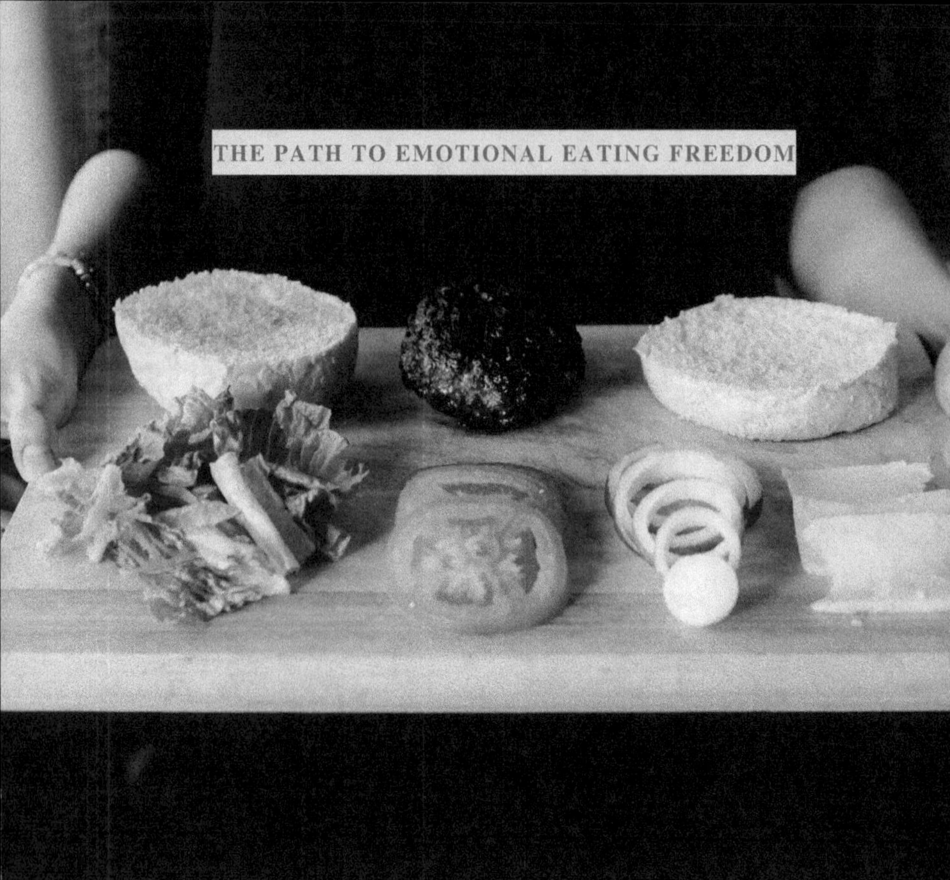

BITE. CHEW. SWALLOW.

One of the problems in our daily lives is that many of us rush through the day, with no time for anything … and when we have time to get a bite to eat, we gobble it down.

That leads to stressful, unhealthy living.

Perhaps you might wonder, why should you eat slowly?

Scientists have known for some time that a full stomach is only part of what causes someone to feel satisfied after a meal; the brain must also receive a series of signals from digestive hormones secreted by the gastrointestinal tract.

Stretch receptors in the stomach are activated as it fills with food or water; these signal the brain directly through the vagus nerve that connects gut and brainstem. Hormonal signals are released as partially digested food enters the small intestine. One example is cholecystokinin (CCK), released by the intestines in response to food consumed during a meal. Another hormone, leptin, produced by fat cells, is an adiposity signal that communicates with the brain about long-range needs and satiety, based on the body's energy stores.

Research suggests that leptin amplifies the CCK signals, to enhance the feeling of fullness. Other research suggests that leptin also interacts with the neurotransmitter dopamine in the brain to produce a feeling of pleasure after eating. The theory is that, by eating too quickly, people may not give this intricate hormonal cross-talk system enough time to work.

Of course, as anyone who has tried eating slowly in order to lose weight can attest, it's not quite that simple. People who are obese, for example, may suffer from leptin resistance, meaning that they are less responsive to satiety or pleasure signals from this hormone. People are also sensitive to cues in the environment — such as the alluring smell of chocolate chip cookies or the sight of a juicy burger — that can trigger the desire to eat.

Are there benefits to eating slowly?

The benefits of slow eating include better digestion, better hydration, easier weight loss or maintenance, and greater satisfaction with our meals. Meanwhile, eating quickly leads to poor digestion, increased weight gain, and lower satisfaction.

 **Solution**

While it may seem intuitive that a "quick bite" would cause us to eat less, mindless speed-eating actually does the opposite: We eat more. It's possible to correct your speed-eating habits by making a handful of simple changes.

- **Ground your mind.** Grounding techniques are a powerful way to support yourself through heavy emotional times. They help to bring you back to the present moment, preventing you from being swept away by your feelings and resorting to mindlessly eating. One way you can ground your mind is by either taking a moment to close your eyes, breathe, notice your heart rate, your breathing, and how you feel. Think of two happy moments that happened to you throughout the day which you are thankful for.

- **Chew each bite 20 or more times.** This simple-sounding tip is tougher than you might think. The trick is to be mindful, purposeful and tenacious. Chewing slowly will help you reduce the amount of food you eat (or times you overeat) and improve gastrointestinal hormone responses as well. In fact, a 2011 study found that extra chewing significantly reduced calorie intake and lowered plasma levels of ghrelin, the hormone that tells you to eat more.

- **Pay attention to volume.** Measuring out portions or even using your fist as a rough guideline and choosing small plates to help with portion control helps with developing mindful eating habits.

- **Eat at a table, without distractions** like the television. If you want to connect with those in your household, eat slower, and improve your health and your children's food choices, try family dinners at a table with no distractions (eg: TV or mobile phones).

- **Savor the flavor.** Think about the food you're eating and the healthful ingredients in it. The more real, whole foods you eat, the more you'll be able to savor your healthy, tasty choices. Thinking through ingredients often makes you want to choose nourishing ones and omit foods with chemicals and junk ingredients. Who wants to spend their dinner thinking about Blue dye #20 or some other chemical name that you can't pronounce?

- **Make it a bit tougher.** Ever wonder why some people tend to overeat less than others? Or even why children take so long to eat? Our utensils have made the whole "shoveling" food habit a little too easy. Instead, make it tougher (using utensils is hard for kids). Try chopsticks; you'll likely eat slower.

- While slowing down, **make yourself aware of how full you are (or aren't)**. When you start to feel full, put down your fork, wait a few minutes, and then decide if you really want more or not. If you are part of the "clean-plate" club, save your leftovers for lunch. The next time, give yourself smaller portions. If needed, have a glass of water, sit for five minutes, and then decide if you want more.

- **Keep the extras in the kitchen.** Family-style dinner service (like the picture above), in which all the foods are on the table and passed around is fun, but should be reserved for special occasions. For everyday dinners, fill your plate and then take it to the table, while leaving any extra behind in the kitchen. You'll be less likely to dig into unintended "seconds" if you have to get up and walk to another room to get them.

121 | TIP #12 DEHYDRATION HUNGER

"

IF THERE IS MAGIC ON THIS PLANET, IT IS CONTAINED IN WATER.

LOREN EISELEY

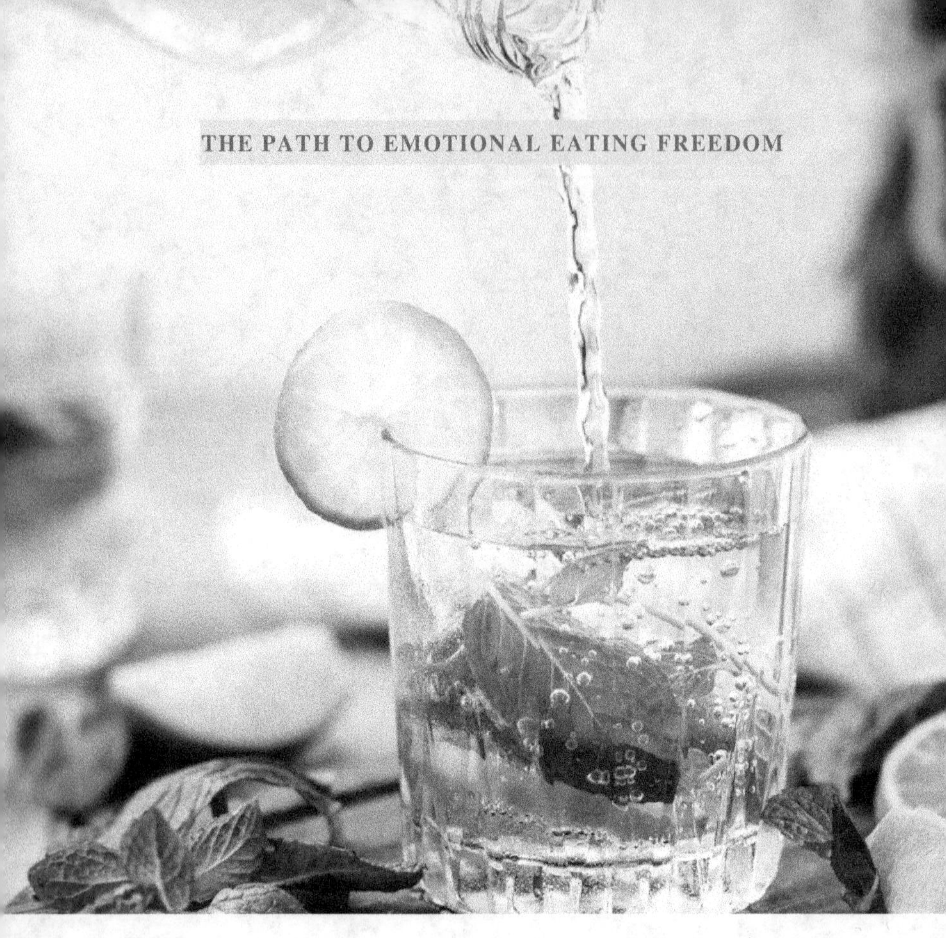

THE POWER OF WATER

Overeating isn't something that just happens, we all have reasons for doing it. Sometimes those reasons are emotional or mental, but sometimes they're purely physical. Surprisingly, dehydration is one of the main causes of overeating - and it is sneaky. We call it "dehydration hunger."

Read on to understand why dehydration hunger

could be tricking your body into some unhealthy eating habits – and adding on those extra pounds.

Reason #1: Dehydration makes you think you're hungry

One of the most baffling tricks your body plays on your brain is that it tends to disguise dehydration as hunger. Often, you may think you're craving a tasty snack when in fact your body is calling out for H20. Why the mind games? It has to do with the liver not getting enough water, and not being able to produce glycogens, which give you that energized, full feeling. Low glycogen count means plenty of trips to the fridge—and could mean a higher number on the scale.

Reason #2: Dehydration zaps your energy

Dehydration is one of the leading causes of fatigue. When you don't get enough water, hundreds of biological processes in your body lack support, and your organs have to work much harder to do their jobs—making you tired and weak. Consequently, your blood pressure drops, which sends the signal to your brain that it's time to raid the snack cabinet.

Crafty, huh? It's a steep downward spiral, and it all starts when you don't drink enough water.

Reason #3: Dehydration makes you crave…salt?!

In another bizarre bit of biological trickery, your brain sometimes misinterprets thirst as the need for salt. Dehydrated bodies actually crave sodium—a nutrient that can dehydrate it even further! What a vicious cycle!

This one has a simpler explanation: when we sweat (which we do all day, every day, regardless of whether we feel it or not), we lose vital salts as well as water.

According to researchers, approximately 3 out of 4 Americans are chronically dehydrated, which means you most likely need to be drinking more water than you are.

 **Solution**

If you're struggling to shed some pounds, or find yourself eating more than you should, dehydration hunger may be the culprit.

Try making it a habit to drink water (1-2 cups) *before* eating. Doing this can make you feel more full, which can help with restraint during mealtimes. Plus, eliminating phantom hunger, exhaustion, and the craving for salty foods will give you a leg up on your overeating habits.

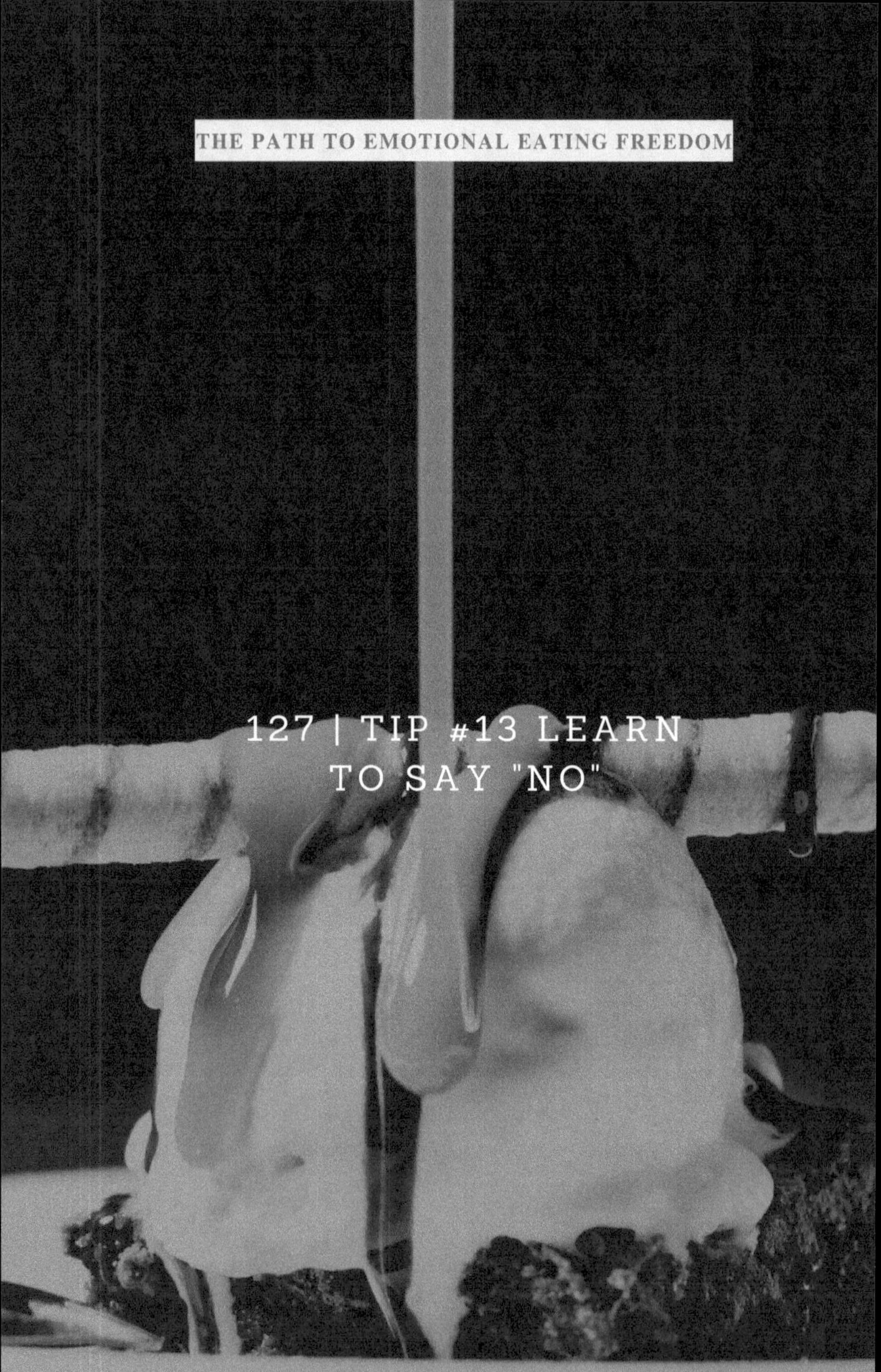

127 | TIP #13 LEARN TO SAY "NO"

HALF OF THE TROUBLES OF THIS LIFE CAN BE TRACED TO SAYING YES TOO QUICKLY AND NOT SAYING NO SOON ENOUGH.

JOSH BILLINGS

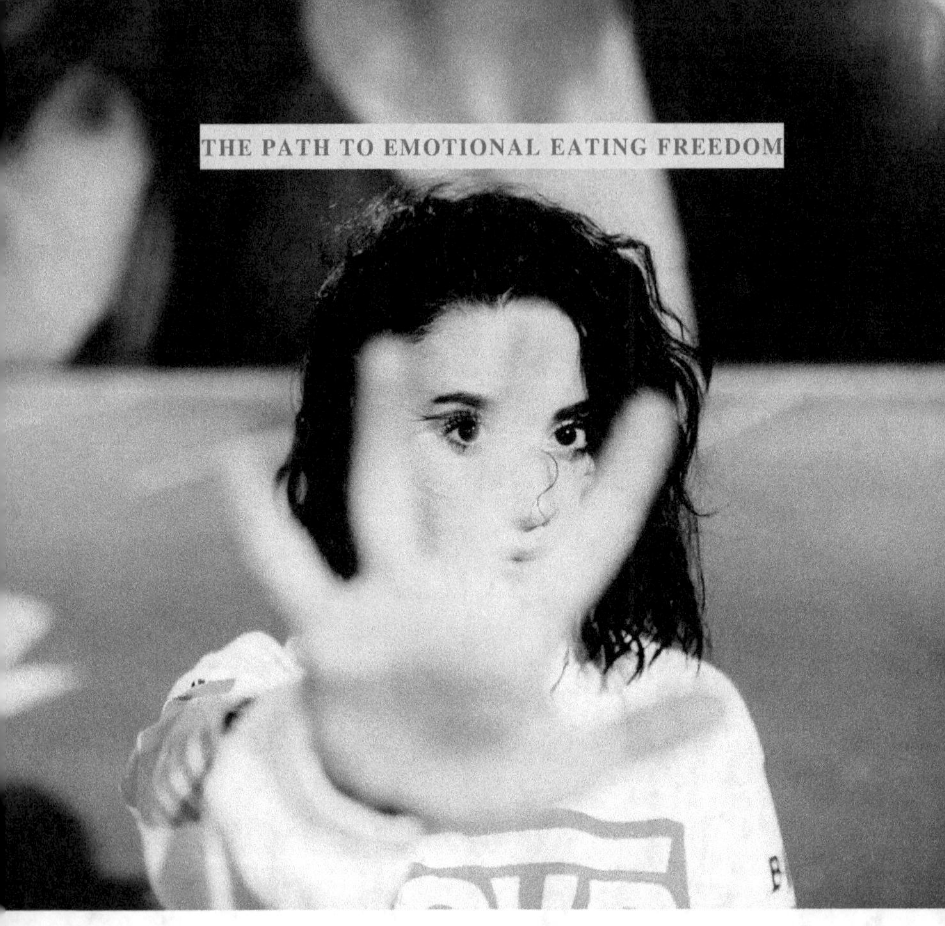

STAND UP FOR YOUR OWN WELL-BEING

Let's be honest, we like to be liked. And one way to try to paint ourselves in a favorable light with others is by saying "yes" to their requests, regardless of how many plates we are already trying to spin.

If you're wondering what this had to do with why you can't stop overeating…

Have you heard the saying "you can't pour from an empty cup?" Well, you can't expect a woman who runs from dusk to dawn managing kids, a home, and all those people-pleasing responsibilities to have much left in the tank to say "no" to those sugary sweets.

Another scenario why learning how to say "no" is truly a much needed skill to start practicing is because sometimes we avoid saying "no" to a friend, family or colleague who offers us a delicious snack because we don't want to hurt their feelings?

Maybe it is a loved one's anniversary or a colleague's birthday and someone baked a mountain full of delicious muffins and cookies to celebrate the occasion. Though people may offer you to dig in out of love and kindness, but if you are full, you are full. Why must you feel bad and eat more than you really want to simply because you are worried you will hurt the feelings of others?

Then what about *your* feelings? Don't they matter?

You'd rather be angry with yourself for overeating than to politely reject someone's offer to eat more after you've already reached your limit?

Not respecting your need for rest, quiet, relaxation, and trying to please others can lead to making disrespectful choices towards your body.

 **Solution**

Saying no doesn't have to be as hard or as complicated as we make it. You can use a few simple strategies to strengthen your no muscle and when you do this you'll add more ease to your life and eliminate pounds of stress.

Step #1 Respect your desire to be kind, and start by making a positive statement. Examples might be, "I'm so honored that you asked me", "Thank you so much for thinking of me", "It sounds like a very important project" or "It's so sweet of you to offer me these mouth-watering treats."

Step #2 Next, make your no a simple statement. The easiest way to say no, even though it's difficult at first, is to keep it short and sweet, with little elaboration or comment. Some examples are phrases like "I'm sorry I can't", "It just won't work for me", "Unfortunately I'm unable to", "Forgive me, my stomach just can't take in anymore" or simply, "I just can't eat anymore."

Step #3 Deliver the message in a pleasant tone of voice and then stop talking. If you have difficulty saying no, you've probably experienced a situation when you started by saying no and ended up explaining or discussing your reasons until they turned into a yes. Staying silent after you've said no is the most challenging part of this formula. Alternatively, if you feel an awkward moment arising, you can politely excuse yourself to make a phone call or go to the toilet.

If you ever come across someone who is really pushy and tries to shove food down your throat (believe me, I've met a few), then the only way to make yourself heard in such times is to have even more courage to stand up for yourself and say in a clear, assertive tone, "No, thank you very much. I'll pass for now."

Is there a possibility you might offend or hurt the other person?

Maybe.

But as I said earlier, you can't please everyone.

Imagine you were really full after a good meal and 10 different people that you know offered you 2 muffins each, would you accept and eat all the 20 muffins just because you feel bad?

Are you going to force feed yourself like a goose just because you are worried you might hurt someone's feelings?

There is a time for being a little more giving and then there is a time to be realistic if giving is possible or not, taking into consideration whether to please others will be at the expense of your own health and mental well-being.

In these kinds of scenarios, is exactly the time to stand up for yourself and do what's right by you.

134 | TIP #14 KEEP YOUR MOUTH MINTY-FRESH

"

MINDFULNESS ISN'T DIFFICULT, WE JUST NEED TO REMEMBER TO DO IT.

SHARON SALZBERG

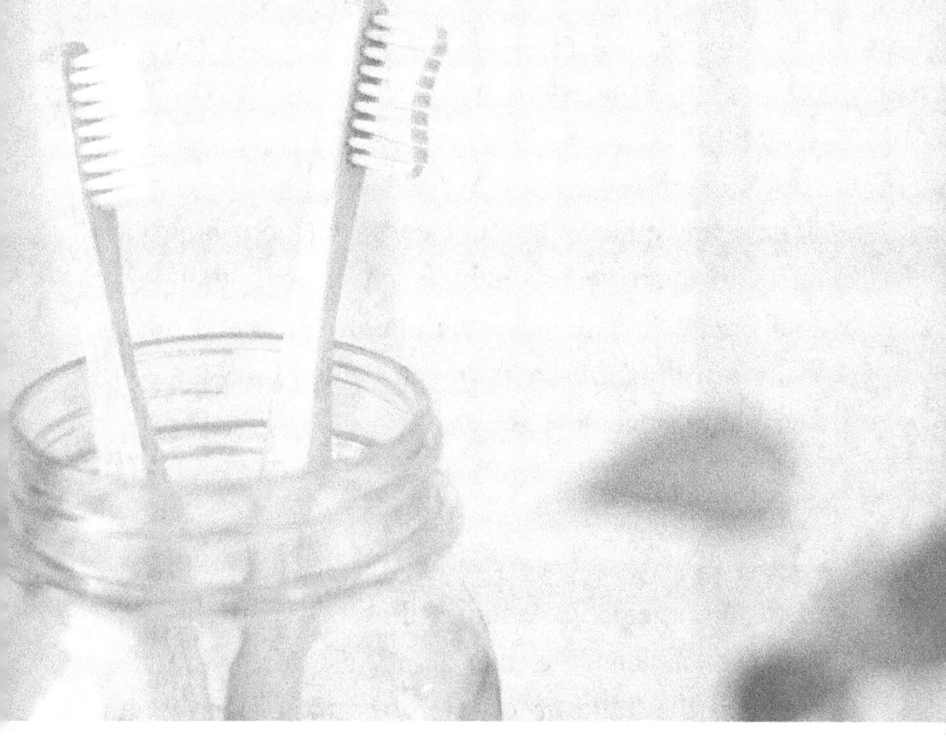

THE BEST UNDERUSED TRICK

You've probably gulped a glass of orange juice in the morning, right after brushing your teeth and it didn't taste so good, right? Brushing your teeth after you're done eating has that effect with more than just orange juice.

Once your mouth feels minty-fresh, food and drink

will not be *that* palatable, so you're more likely to skip them. Your mouth and your waistline will thank you for it.

There are quite a few evidences that brushing can help to keep your weight in check and limit your calorie intake, yes the latter claim is true and this is why brushing can help you in being real with your weight management goals.

How does it help?

Brushing helps to remove the food particles and plaques attached to the gums and teeth and this reduces the build-up of microbes that can mix with the saliva and play tricks with the brain to induce a feeling of hunger. In fact, a good way to keep your munchies at bay is to always brush your teeth when you're itching for a snack that you know you shouldn't eat. Not only will brushing your teeth make you forget that guilt-pleasure, but it will also help you keep your mouth fresh and free of bad breath.

Probably this is a reason why toothpicks are such a favourite with people who are on a diet.

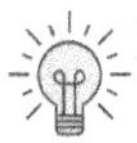 **Solution**

If you are someone who normally brushes your teeth once or twice daily and also has taken up weight loss goals seriously, then try upping the number of times you brush in a day. Try brushing your teeth once during your lunch break, in-between your meals or before having an evening snack.

This might cut down on your cravings and also help you to pick healthier options than the fat food variants.

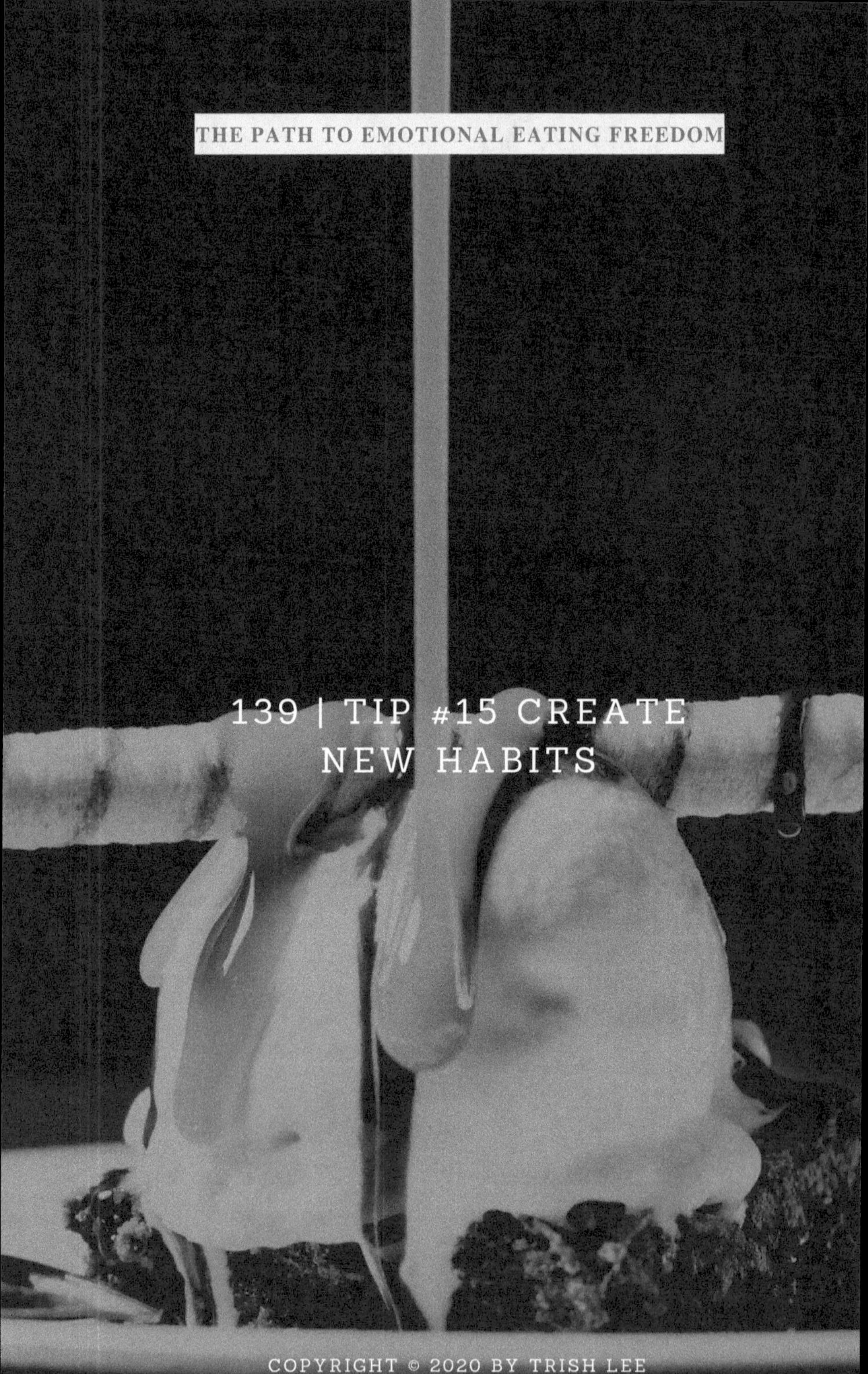

139 | TIP #15 CREATE NEW HABITS

"

DEPENDING ON WHAT THEY ARE, OUR HABITS WILL EITHER MAKE US OR BREAK US. WE BECOME WHAT WE REPEATEDLY DO.

SEAN COVEY

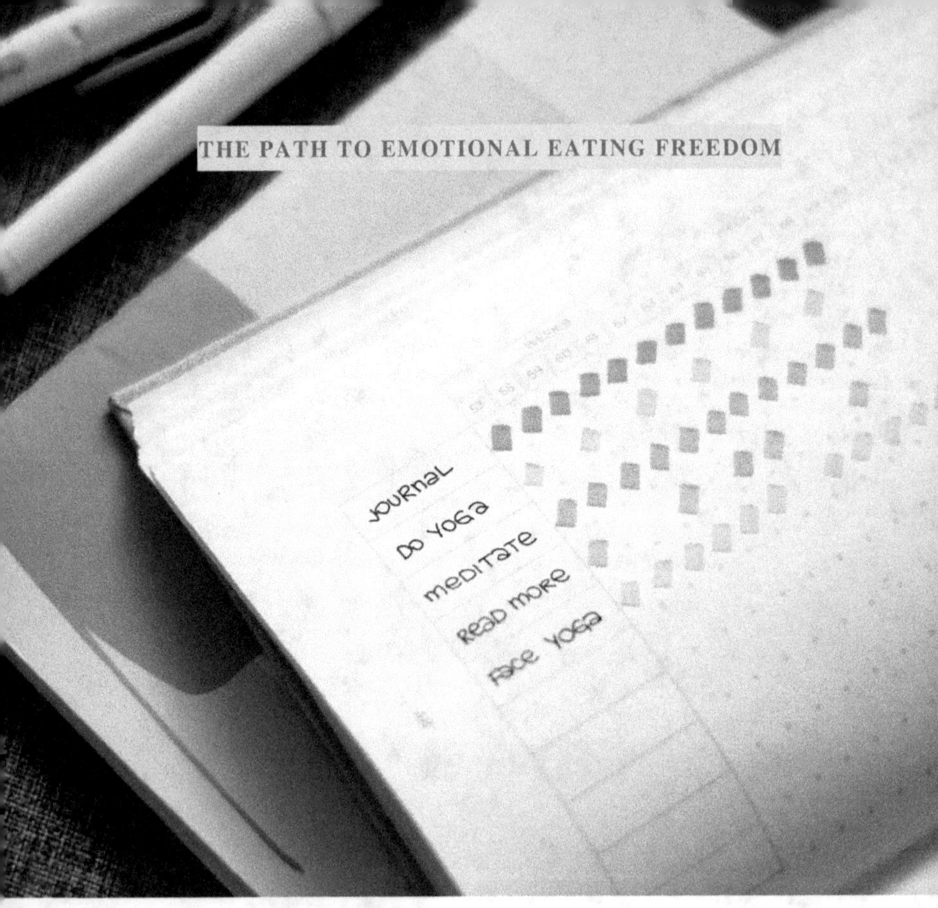

PRACTICE HABITS THAT SERVE YOU

Many of us have developed the not-so-good habit of getting home, putting down our stuff, and immediately heading to the kitchen to bury our feelings in cookies, soft drinks, cake or leftover pasta.

It is understandable that after a long day, a nice warm lasagna or creamy chocolate lava cake can seem very tempting.

 **Solution**

Create a new homecoming habit. As soon as you reach home, remove your shoes, put aside your belongings, and say out loud, "I leave my troubles here." Next, replace the customary trip to the kitchen with a non-food activity that brings you pleasure, such as:

- Hugging your partner
- Playing with your child
- Putting on music
- Hugging your dog or cat
- Writing in your diary about your day or journal about the people or things you are grateful for
- Enjoying your comfy sofa
- Admiring the view from a window or water your plants.

Once you are more relaxed and centered, you can then make a more mindful decision if you really are hungry and how much you need to eat to nourish your body.

Do this every day for a few weeks, and you're well on your way to building a new ritual.

143 | TIP #16 OUT OF SIGHT, OUT OF MIND

"

OUT OF SIGHT,
OUT OF MIND.
IT'S HOW I COPE.

LISA RENEE JONES

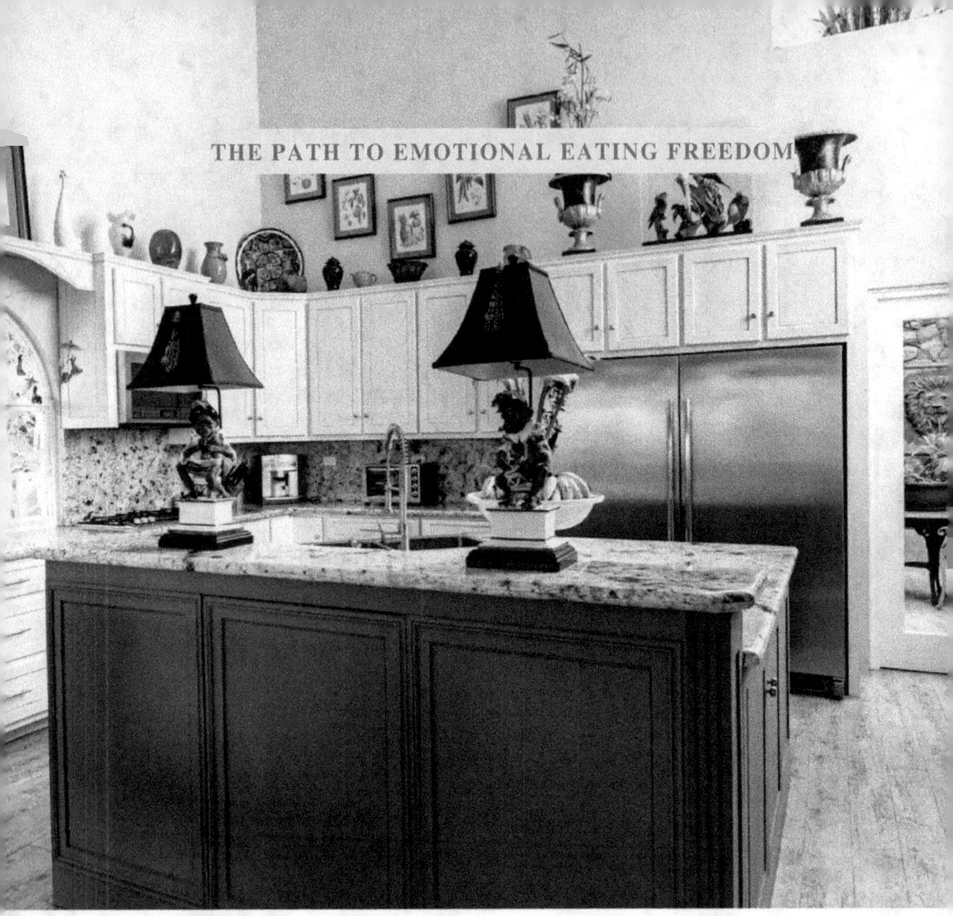

TEMPT NOT, WANT NOT

As if dealing with emotional issues isn't hard enough, having junk food displayed in easy-to-reach places makes the temptation to just sink your teeth into a nice crunchy cookie even harder to deny.

 **Solution**

Take common offenders out of your pantry or hide them in a less visible corner of your kitchen.

Try not to keep junk food in your home. Your brain is going to seek out junk food, so why would you put yourself in the easy situation to indulge in it?

Consider trashing or donating foods in your cupboards that you often reach for in moments of strife. Think high-fat, sweet or calorie-laden things, like chips, chocolate, and ice cream. Another trick you can try is instead of giving away food, hide all these goodies in a hard to reach storage cabinet (to be opened on special occasions). Also postpone trips to the grocery store when you're feeling upset.

Keeping the foods you crave out of reach when you're feeling emotional may help break the cycle by giving you time to think before noshing.

Step into your kitchen, look around... What do you see? Are your favourite snacks in plain sight or in easy-to-reach places? If yes, start reorganising your kitchen to make it less tempting to support your journey toward creating a healthier life for yourself.

147 | TIP #17 CREATE A SCHEDULE

PROFESSIONALS STICK TO THE SCHEDULE; AMATEURS LET LIFE GET IN THE WAY.

JAMES CLEAR

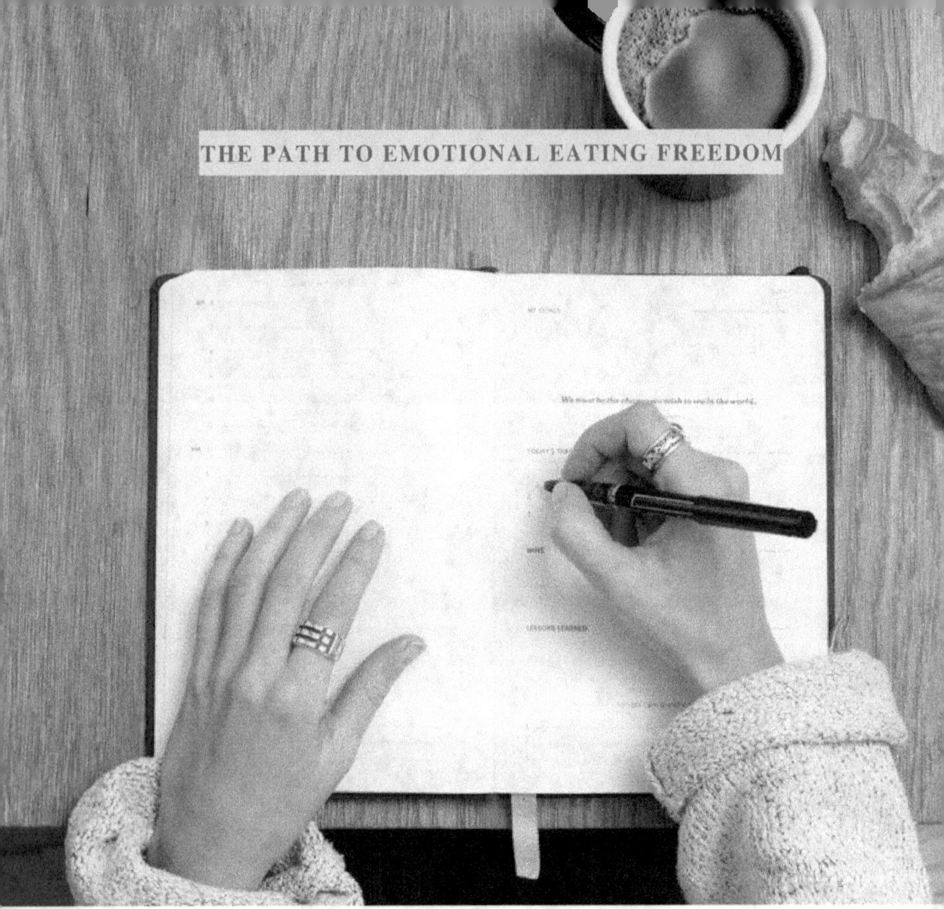

DEVELOP A SET EATING SCHEDULE

Settling into a consistent routine will help regulate blood sugar and insulin levels, hunger hormones, mental and physical energy, digestive health, and even your sleep cycle. On the other hand, irregular eating habits usually spell trouble because they result in random eating and overeating.

 **Solution**

Real hunger usually kicks in starting about three hours after your last meal. Depending on your eating habits and the time of day, a small snack may be sufficient at that point; if not, you're getting a signal that it's time for your next meal.

Similar to finding a diet plan that suits you best (refer to tip #10), knowing how many meals in a day you need to keep you feeling your best also requires a little trial and error as well as learning how to tune in into your body's needs.

For example, I find having a small dessert right after lunch is fine and doesn't make me feel too sluggish after I'm done. Where else if I eat snacks a few hours after lunch (or what some would call 'coffee time'), I find myself super stuffed and end up not being able to eat a proper nutritious dinner.

Again, don't listen too much to what other people say you should do or what magazines recommend about the number of meals to have in a day, find a routine that gives you the optimum level of energy throughout the day and stick to it as best as you can every day. Consistency is the key to success.

A Gentle note:

Depending on your level of activity in a day, the amount of food you need for energy *will* vary. Not only that, our body's metabolism changes as we age. This is also an important point not to forget. Because the amount of food your body needs will also change accordingly. No 70 year old person can eat the same way as when they were 17 years old.

Pay mindful attention to your body's needs and eat accordingly. Eat when you need to. Don't restrict or deprive your body of its needs.

152 | TIP #18 LOVED UP, POUNDS UP

"

TAKE CARE OF YOUR BODY. IT'S THE ONLY PLACE YOU HAVE TO LIVE.

JIM ROHN

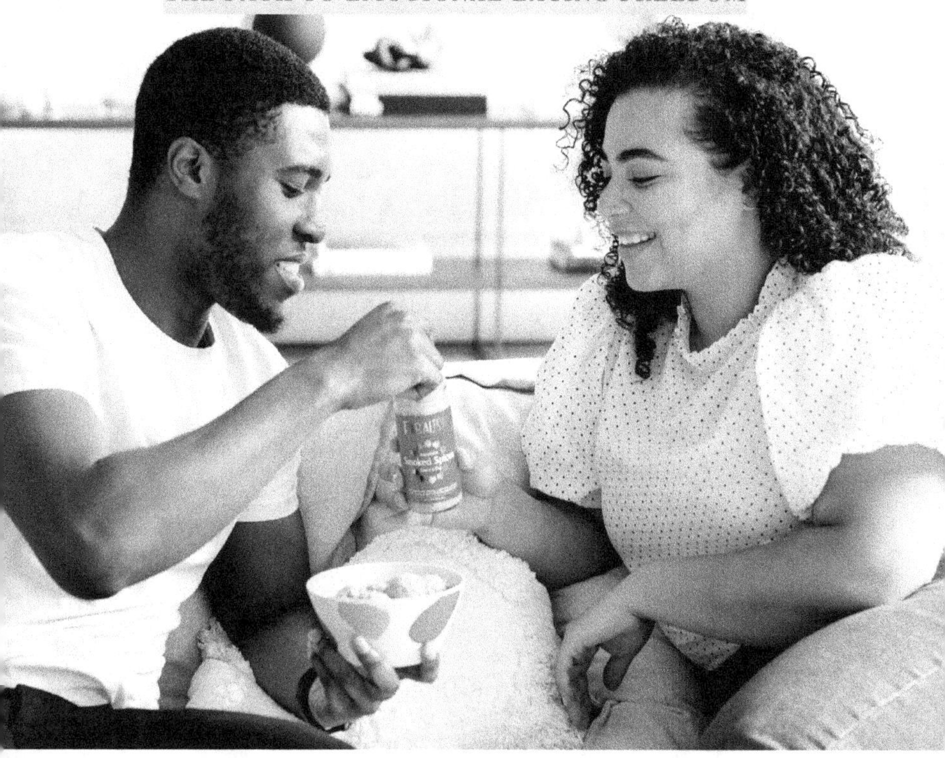

BUTTERFLIES (AND JUNK) IN MY STOMACH...

Falling in love is beautiful, but strangely enough, why do we tend to fall out of love with ourselves and let ourselves go after we've fallen in love?

Men and women without disordered eating issues tend to put on weight when they're coupled up. A 2018 survey of 2,000 Americans found that 69%

of the men and 45% of the women gained weight when getting into their most recent relationship, mostly due to eating out more and moving around less, preferring to cozy up on the couch. A different study followed 169 newlywed couples for four years and found that the happier they were together, the more pounds they gained.

In fact, researchers agree that the most satisfying and happy relationships promote greater weight gain, while marital problems and divorces around the corner often result in weight loss.

Why does love make you fat?

Falling in love doesn't automatically make you gain weight per se. The reasons for this weight gain are different. The researchers point out that in many cases this is because people adapt to the other's living habits, which are not always the healthiest.

In the case of women it was seen that they tend to eat more foods high in fat and sugars, developing a distortion in the perception of portion sizes, which leads them to eat the same amount as their male partners, not realizing that the caloric requirements for men is not the same for women. In fact, some of the women surveyed admitted to have eaten the same amount as their male partners or even more.

It was also noted that couples tend to spend more time and effort in preparation of meals. If we live alone it is likely we skip a few meals or snack something quick, but living in pairs we tend to prepare more lavish dinners, with dessert or alcohol included. In married life, meals have a more important role because they are also the moments when we get together.

In addition, it is normal that we want to spend more time with each other in a relationship, which can cause some people to abandon or neglect exercising and slip slowly into a less active lifestyle. When priorities change, we dedicate less time to personal care.

In fact, the researchers saw that couples who grow fat tend to follow a pattern: after the period of the first meetings, when both frequented bars and restaurants, the relationship gets solid and they decide to live together, they tend to organize larger dinners and spend weekends at home, watching movies and eating popcorn or ice cream on the couch. Obviously, this passive lifestyle is the cause of weight gain.

A study done by the New England Journal of Medicine showed that weight gain is also contagious in married couples. If one partner is gaining weight, the other partner has a 37% chance of gaining more weight as well.

 **Solution**

It is vital to influence each other in positive ways with healthy eating habits and lifestyles regardless of weight in order to enjoy each other's company for the rest of your lives.

Why?

Because if you love someone, don't you wish to have as much time as possible with them? Meaning, to live a long life together. If one or both of you start to spiral into an overeating fiesta, chances are, you'll increase the risk of getting health issues down the road.

Imagine this, if both you and your partner have

chronic sicknesses in your senior years, both of you will have to use a lot of time and energy worrying and looking after each other rather than having happy moments together.

Love and respect yourself enough to influence your partner to eat mindfully with you. Practice expressing love and happiness in other ways other than food (refer to tip #9).

159 | TIP #19 THE BATTLE TO CHANGE: PAIN VS PLEASURE

NOT EVERYTHING THAT IS FACED CAN BE CHANGED, BUT NOTHING CAN BE CHANGED UNTIL IT IS FACED.

JAMES BALDWIN

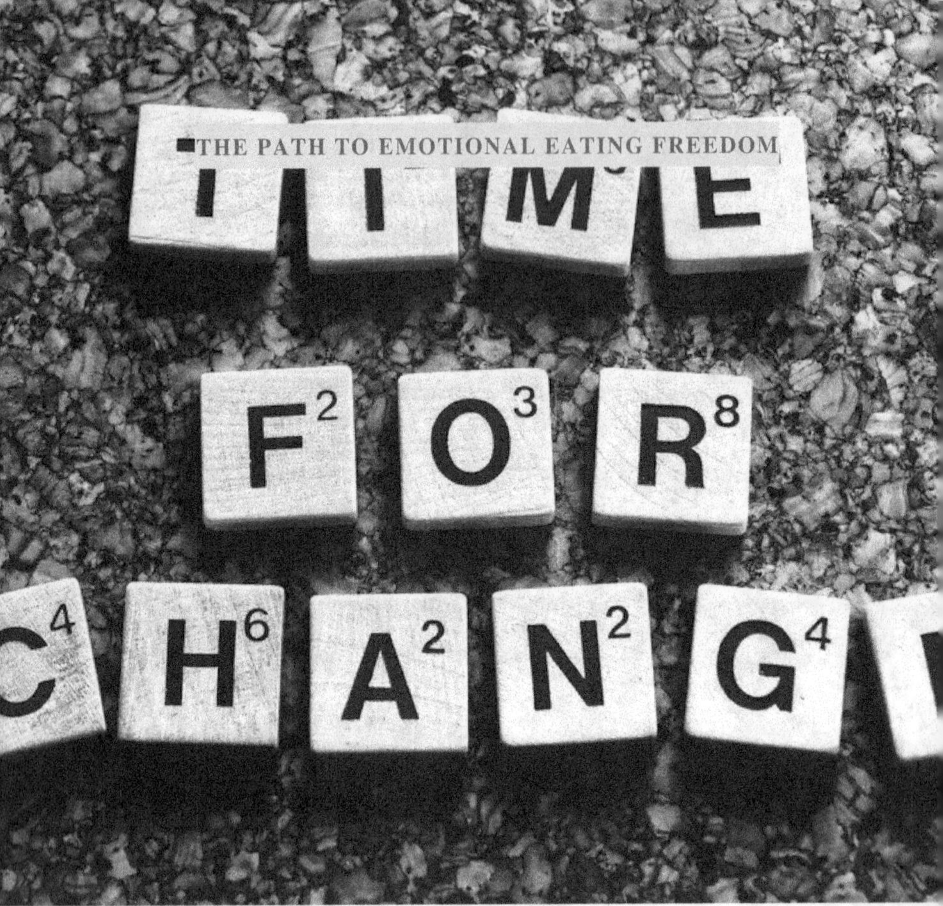

I GIVE UP!

Change, transformation, alteration … however one may choose to name it, can be seen all around us. Whether it's making healthier lifestyle choices, or deciding to be a little more friendly to that colleague at work; more often than not, we all have personal behaviors we wish we could adjust, stop, or start. From a young age we are introduced to change, some more often than others, and somewhere along the line we begin to form our own perceptions on the subject.

The mere mention of the word "change" may cause some to feel uneasy. We often find ourselves resisting change, perhaps because of the perceived risk or fear associated with it. This resistance can be seen in students who always finds himself or herself procrastinating, the 10-year smoker who keeps having "one more," or the overly stressed boss who continues to add to his plate. It's an interesting predicament we put ourselves in. So why do we have such a hard time initiating or following through with our desire to change?

A renowned psychologist, James Prochaska, proposed that we often find ourselves in the previously described predicaments as a result of our perception of change.

He shares that there are 5 stages to change:
1. Pre-contemplation
2. Contemplation
3. Preparation

4. Action stage
5. Maintenance stage

Stage 1 Pre-Contemplation

The first stage of change is one in which individuals may be aware of the behavioral change they desire; however, they have no conscious intention of altering, changing, or stopping their behavior. Often times this may be due to a lack of insight or full awareness into their problems.

Stage 2 Contemplation

The contemplation stage of change is characterized by having further insight and awareness into the behavior that is up for debate. At this stage, an individual acknowledges that they have a problem and begins an internal debate about pursuing change. This can be the most difficult and frustrating stage of change, as it entails a high level of uncertainty. A substantial amount of time may be spent in this stage because many people may not find themselves ready to commit to making a change. They may remain in this stage, perhaps feeling "stuck" as they go back and forth between measuring the benefits and costs of behavioral change.

 **Solution**

To progress through the contemplation stage — and perhaps rid yourself of the overwhelming sense of uncertainty — it may be helpful to do a cost and benefit analysis. Conduct a thorough analysis of the advantages and disadvantages of continuing with the proposed behavior or moving forward with behavioral change. The most helpful way to do this might be to actually sit down with a **pen and paper** and write your thoughts out (note: Writing helps give you more clarity).

BONUS TIP! The reason why many people fail to change is because they attach more pleasure (positive points) to not changing and more pain (negative points) toward change. Therefore, if you are determined to make a change, flip it around, attach more pleasure to change and more pain to not changing, see the magic of change happen faster than you can blink.

Example

Behavior Up for Debate: Emotional eating

Advantages of Continuing: Stress relief, snack breaks

Disadvantages of Continuing: Not good for my health, expensive, overweight, low self-esteem, fiance upset with me

Advantages of Changing: Improve health, improve relationships, more self-confidence, more self-love, save money

Disadvantages of Continuing: Might miss having the outlet for stress relief

After outlining the pros and cons of the change in mind and you decide to proceed to go with the change because you realize that the pros outweigh the cons, then you are ready to move into the Preparation stage.

Stage 3 Preparation

Individuals progress to the preparation stage of change upon committing to the intention to change in the immediate future. The advantages of making said change have been established as outweighing the costs that they might incur. It is at this stage that one may begin to actually take or experiment with small steps towards change, typically within a period of one month. For example, someone who would like to eat healthier may purchase a nutritious eating cookbook.

In this stage, one must develop a detailed plan for contingencies in order to stay on track.
For example: If my behavioral change is to quit emotional eating, what will I do if a friend offers me a slice of pie when I'm already full? (Answer: Refer to tip #13)

Positive reinforcement from others — such as someone treating you to a movie after your first week of successful behavioral change — as well as from yourself — getting a massage or pedicure, say, after two weeks of success — may help you through the progression of this stage. Be sure to share your commitment and plans for change with friends and family and encourage them to follow up with you in regards to your progress.

Stage 4 Action Stage
When individuals move from planning to doing they progress to the action stage of change. Someone within this stage has put his or her plans into action and made significant behavioral changes within the past one to six months. By adhering to our plans, we

have made substantial adjustments to our relationships, routines, environments, and perhaps even to ourselves in order to further the change we desire to achieve.

For example, someone looking to decrease procrastination may have begun to keep and follow a realistic and purposeful daily schedule.

Stage 5 Maintenance Stage

In the maintenance stage, your once desired behavior is now a reality and has been for the past six months. An individual may come to realize that the one thing they doubted they could do is actually possible. Your new behavior is firmly established and the threat of returning to old behaviors becomes less intense or frequent.

Out of all the stages, this stage is by far the most important. It is through this stage that an individual will work towards sustaining long-term change. The possibility of relapsing to old behaviors and re-cycling through the stages may always be present, so it's important to continue planning for events that might trigger your old behaviors to reappear.

What you can try is, recalling what helped you through previous stages, such as a cost and benefit analysis. This can help during this stage when you feel less strong.

Bottom line is, change *is* possible. With a little planning, a little dedication, and a dash of faith in yourself, you can definitely make any change that you set your mind to.

Ready to make a change? I'm betting you are. That's why you got this book in the first place. Don't stop now! You're already in Stage 2 (Contemplation). Write out clearly what is the desired change you'd like to make and what is the envisioned outcome.

Draw a line down the middle. One side will be the pros, the other side the cons.

Be completely honest with yourself and write out all the pros and cons that you can expect to experience as a result of the change that you want. Once ready, move on to the next stage and make that change a reality.

You got this!

169 | TIP #20 LONELINESS & LOW SELF-ESTEEM

66

LACK OF CONFIDENCE IS WHAT MAKES YOU WANT TO CHANGE SOMEBODY ELSE'S MIND. WHEN YOU'RE OK, YOU DON'T NEED TO CONVINCE ANYONE ELSE IN ORDER TO EMPOWER YOURSELF.

JADA PINKETT SMITH

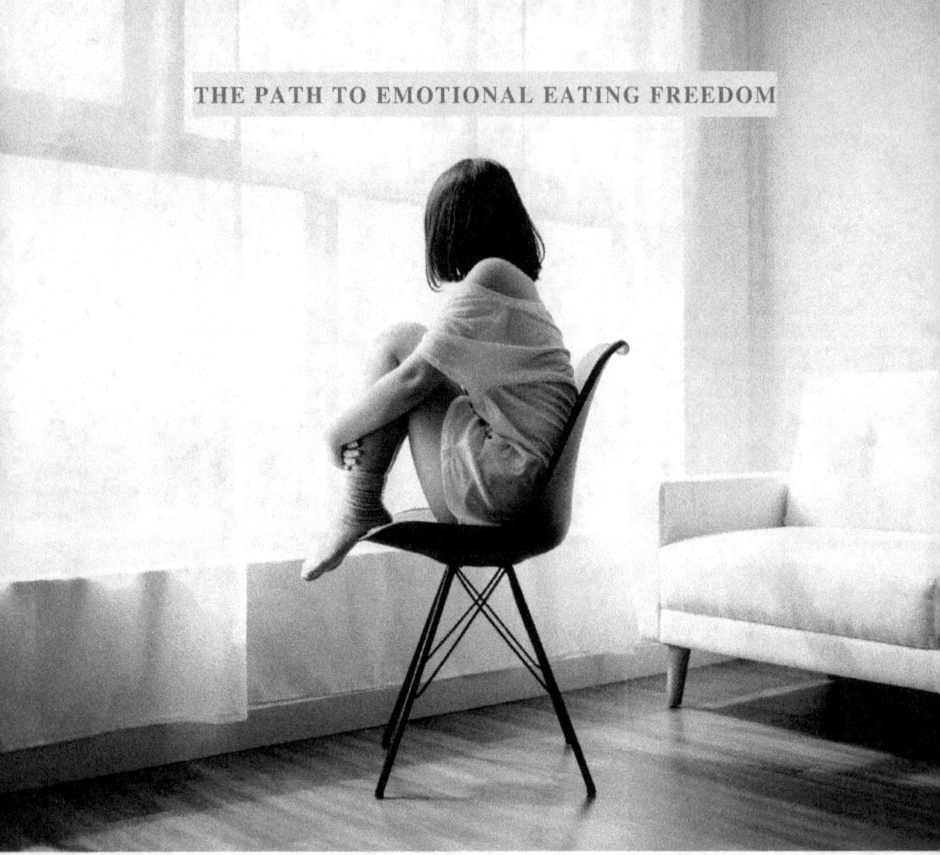

NO ONE LIKES ME...

It is common for many people, especially young people to feel increasingly uncomfortable with their bodies as changes occur during adolescence. Low self-esteem occurs when expectations of how you want your body to look don't match up to reality. These types of feelings can lead to distorted thoughts and emotions about your bodies and negative thoughts about body image and self-worth can lead to changes in eating (eating disorder) and exercise behaviors.

Battling with low self-esteem and loneliness was the main reason that lead me to my unhealthy emotional eating (aka. eating disorder) habit.

What is an eating disorder?

Eating disorders usually begin in the late teenage years, but can start at any age and continue into adulthood. Eating disorders are usually related to emotional issues such as control and self-esteem. They are often a way of avoiding thinking about the real problems. There are usually a number of factors that contribute to them. These can be things that have happened to you, such as difficult relationships with friends or family, physical, emotional or sexual abuse, loss and grief, stress, or feeling that you've lost control over life.

Types of eating disorders

1. **Anorexia nervosa** is to do with extreme concerns about weight, fear of gaining weight or becoming fat, and deliberately keeping a very

low body weight by deliberately limiting the amount of food eaten or by over-exercising. Although they are usually underweight, people with this condition believe that they are 'fat'.

2. **Bulimia nervosa** is a compulsive cycle of eating large amounts of food and then trying to avoid weight gain (for example by vomiting, using laxatives or exercising excessively).

3. **Binge eating disorder** is about frequently eating large amounts of food, often when not hungry.

So how can I build up my self-esteem?

 **Solution**

Here are my top 9 ways to build up your self-esteem.

1) Help someone

Use your talents, skills and abilities to help others. Give someone direct assistance, share helpful resources or teach someone something they want to learn. Offer something you do well as a gift to someone.

I started volunteering at orphanages and homes for

the mentally challenged since I was 15 years old. Helping others, especially the less fortunate is without a doubt an enriching, humbling, and most definitely - empowering life experience.

You too have the power to help someone *right now* and make a positive difference in this world.

Off the top of your head, who can you think of that you can offer help to?

And remember, no help is ever too insignificant or useless.

2) Self-acceptance

Stop worrying about what others think and start accepting you just as you are. Have you ever seen a flower and thought it was ugly? Have you ever seen 2 flowers look *exactly* the same (it's stem, petals, everything)?

The answer would most probably be no and no.

Everyone is unique in their own way. Why would you want to be like someone else when you were meant to stand out? When you worry about what others will think of you, you are not allowing yourself to feel free to be completely yourself. Make a firm decision to stop worrying about what other people think--begin making choices based on what you want, not what you think others want from you.

3) Read something inspirational

A great way to gain more self-esteem is to read something that lifts you up and makes you feel positive about yourself.

4) Let negative people go

If there are people in your life who are negative-- who have nothing positive to say or who put you down or take advantage of you--do the smart thing and let them go. The only way to find your self-esteem is to surround yourself with supportive positive people who admire you and value you.

Don't ever be afraid to let people go. You don't *need* someone in order to function or to feel whole. You were born whole.

5) Welcome failure as part of growth

It's a common response to be hard on yourself when you've failed. But if you can shift your thinking to understand that failure is an opportunity to learn, that it plays a necessary role in learning and growth, it can help you keep perspective. Remember too that failure means you're making an effort.

6) Always remain a student

Think of yourself as a lifelong learner. Approach everything that you do with a student's mentality-- what Zen Buddhists call Shoshin or "beginner's mind"--open, eager, unbiased and willing to learn.

7) Heal your past

Unresolved issues and drama can keep you trapped in low self-esteem. Seek the support of a trained counsellor or certified Life Coach to help you heal the past so you can move onto the future in a confident and self-assured way.

8) Draw a line in the sand

The best way to find your self-esteem is to create personal boundaries. Know what your boundaries are and how you wish to respond when people cross them. Don't allow others to control you, take advantage of you or manipulate you. To be confident is to maintain firm boundaries.

9) Dress up

When you look your best, you feel your best. Dress like someone who has confidence and let your self-assurance come through in how you look.

178 | TIP #21 GATHER SUPPORT

> **DON'T BE AFRAID TO ASK QUESTIONS. DON'T BE AFRAID TO ASK FOR HELP WHEN YOU NEED IT. I DO THAT EVERY DAY. ASKING FOR HELP ISN'T A SIGN OF WEAKNESS, IT'S A SIGN OF STRENGTH. IT SHOWS YOU HAVE THE COURAGE TO ADMIT WHEN YOU DON'T KNOW SOMETHING, AND TO LEARN SOMETHING NEW.**

BARACK OBAMA

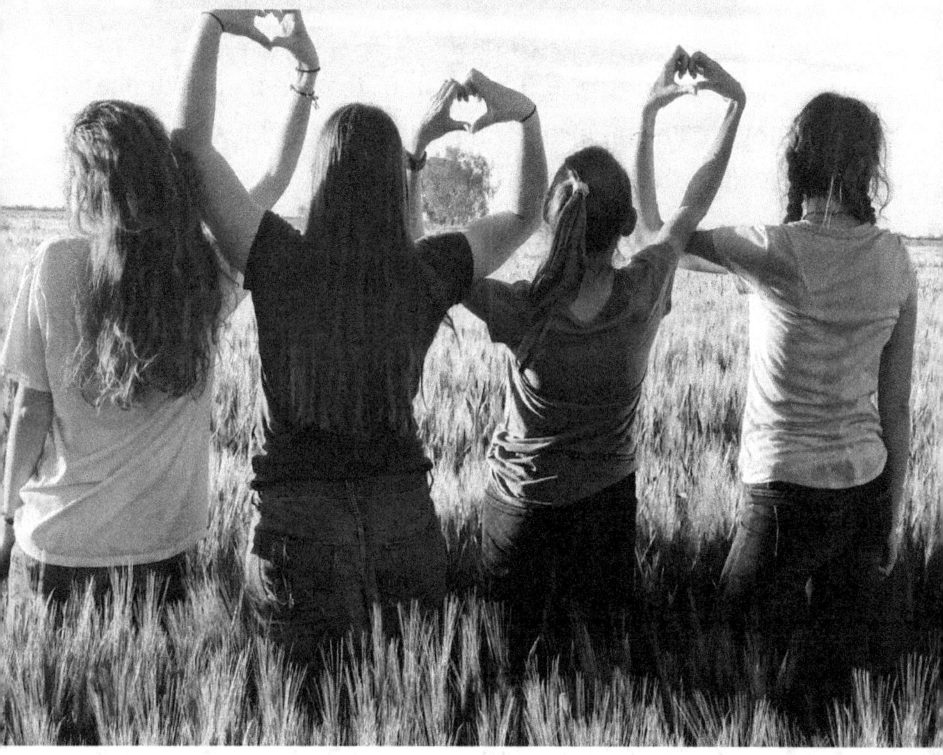

WHAT IF I'M JUDGED?

Some people are afraid to ask for help because they grew up being rather self-sufficient. Their caretakers were not readily available to them. So now as an adult they think that they should not have any needs or wants but only look after others.

Some people feel embarrassed to admit they didn't have all the answers. That might make them look weak or give the impression that the confidence they've been projecting is only a façade. And besides, they should be able to figure it out for themselves. If those comments resonate, you may also suffer from **FOAFH**: Fear of Asking for Help

Part of being a human being is having limitations. No one can do it all. No one. We all need someone. We would literally die without each other.

Why is it important to ask for help?

Everybody has a heavy burden to bear at some point or another, and one of the core purposes of relationships is to help support one another. I once worked with a client who was very hesitant to reach out for help when she needed it. Through therapy, we discovered that this was because growing up she had a weighty responsibility to care for others and believed it was her job to be the person who helps, not the person who needs help. Through understanding her own past, this woman came to understand that as an adult, she no longer needed to rescue the world; she could ask for assistance.

Another reason we shouldn't be afraid to reach out

for help is because complete independence is impossible.

Culturally, we seem to tout independence as this great thing to aspire to, but it's not realistic or even desirable to try to achieve.

As human beings, we are wired to connect with other people. To go against this is to try to defy nature. The goal is healthy interdependence. There's a negotiation of give and take in our relationships. We can't be taking all the time, but trying to only give throws us off balance as well.

Asking for help (in moderation) demonstrates trust and helps build bonds of intimacy in friendships. Exposing your human limitations to someone shows that you're willing to be vulnerable to them.

When we don't ask for help and instead just attempt to do things on our own, we're missing out on an opportunity to build connections with another person. And it can actually be quite a compliment to ask someone else for his or her help. Think about when you've given help before and someone graciously received it. We all want to feel validated in making a difference in someone else's life, and it's a gift to feel like we are needed. Why not share that gift sometimes and ask for a close friend's help?

And finally, we need to get over being afraid of being turned down.

If you ask for someone's help, the worst thing he or she can say is "no"! It doesn't need to be awkward or uncomfortable. I challenge you to not take a "no" answer as a personal rejection. It simply means the other person has limitations (as we all do) and is unable to offer assistance to you at the moment. And that's okay! No need to misinterpret a "no" as meaning that someone doesn't like you or thinks you're unworthy of love. It might sting a little to be told "no" when you ask for help, but try to shake it off and remember that it's not a reflection on you.

 **Solution**

A network of family and friends, including professional help in the form of a therapist or life coach, if necessary, can be as important to your success as your own motivation and efforts.

Surround yourself with people willing to lend an ear,

it could even be cooking, walking or workout buddies to offer you a solid foundation of positive encouragement and motivation.

Those who care about your well-being can help by cheering you on, sharing ideas for healthier meals, recognizing the emotional underpinnings of your overeating issues, and perhaps even helping to diffuse some of the emotional situations that trigger your overeating.

Dealing With A Medical Condition

One last key point that is worth mentioning, if you feel you have a medical condition which is hindering you from losing weight or cause you to experience rapid fluctuations to your weight, please do consult a doctor for professional consultation. Don't be afraid of what the results might be. It could may well be something curable, which means there's absolutely no need to stress about. *If* it is a condition that requires more intensive long-term care from medical professionals, please do what is necessary for your own health.

No matter how intimidating it may be, it is better to deal with it head on and increase your chances of living a healthier and longer life to enjoy this one life you've been blessed with.

Do it for you. You deserve to feel **strong**, **healthy**, and **happy**.

186 | NOW WHAT?

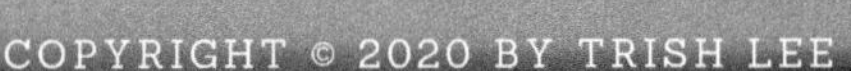

> I COULD ONLY ACHIEVE SUCCESS IN MY LIFE THROUGH SELF-DISCIPLINE, AND I APPLIED IT UNTIL MY WISH AND MY WILL BECAME ONE.

NIKOLA TESLA

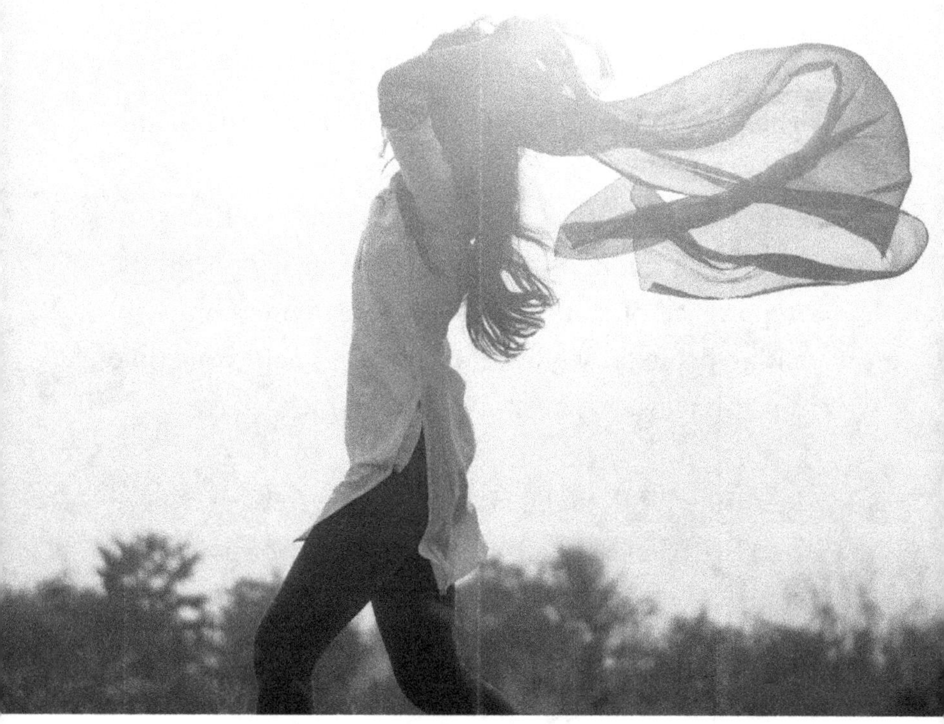

CONGRATULATIONS!

You have now discovered the secrets to emotional mastery and have the tools to enjoy a healthy and fulfilling relationship with food.

Firstly, you learned a deeper understanding on what is emotional eating, the signs of an emotional eater, 3 facts about emotional eaters, how you became an emotional eater, and why it isn't beneficial for your health or mental well-being.

Then we moved on to the most juiciest part of this book and that is you discovered the 21 tips to emotional mastery, how to gain more self-control whenever emotions are clouding your judgment, the importance of self-compassion, create more mindful eating habits as well as mind tools to help you come out stronger whenever you fall off track.

It is truly a gift and a skill to be able to have control over what and how you feed your mind, body, and soul.

Now that you have this wisdom, don't keep it a secret. Tell every one whom you care about that they need not have a love-hate relationship with food. When you come across any friend, family or colleague who is suffering from emotional eating, tell them that with the right coping strategies, they can learn healthier ways to deal with their emotions, avoid triggers, conquer cravings, and share the insights from **The Path To Emotional Eating Freedom** to finally put a stop to their emotional eating.

A last gentle reminder, eating more than you

intended may be distressing. Beating yourself up about it only increases your distress.

If you are feeling discomfort and guilt after a binge, please offer yourself self-compassion and eat the next meal regardless of what you ate earlier. It's okay if you're turning to food more than usual right now to cope. It's okay if you gain weight. You are amazing and still worthy of love.

Practice being kind to yourself. Talk to yourself as you would talk to a close friend or young child you were trying to soothe.

You are not a machine, even machines break down from time to time. Nothing is perfect, so don't put that expectation on yourself. It is ok to fall off track once in awhile, it doesn't mean you are a failure or that all your hard work has been lost. Just accept what's done is done, forgive yourself, and get back on track wiser and stronger each time.

Trust yourself that you are strong and capable to achieve anything you set your mind to.

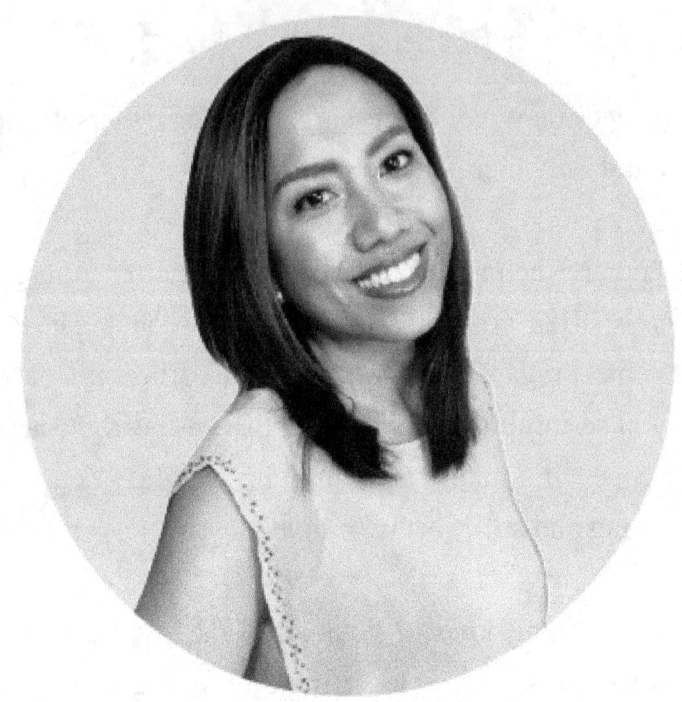

About Trish Lee

Trish's clients include creative professionals, entrepreneurs, and stay-at-home moms who want excellence and well-being in mind, body, and soul.

A born-and-raised girl from Malaysia, Trish is now happily based in Germany with her husband and baby girl.

Through her Life Coaching business, self-help books, and Life-Transforming Programs, Trish continues her life mission of helping others break free from their past to move forward toward shaping a future of their dreams.

Learn more about Trish at **trishandco.com**.

ADDITIONAL RESOURCES

Don't forget to download your free e-book **Rock Solid Self-Confidence For Achievers** to build up your self-esteem, gain more control over your emotions, and to both inspire and help keep you on track with The Path To Emotional Eating Freedom approach.

Visit trishandco.com/ebook-build-unshakeable-confidence now to access this free bonus resource and more.

To learn about Trish's other products and programs, visit trishandco.com.

Chopra, Deepak. *The Seven Spiritual Laws of Success: A Practical Guide to the Fulfillment of Your Dreams.*
Novato, CA: New World Library, 1995.

Kane, Ariel, and Shya Kane. *Working on Yourself Doesn't Work: A Book About Instantaneous Transformation.*
New York: McGraw-Hill, 2009.

Katie, Byron, and Stephen Mitchell. *Loving What Is: Four Questions That Can Change Your Life*. New York: Three Rivers Press, 2003.

Tolle, Eckhart. *The Power of Now: A Guide to Spiritual*
Enlightenment. Novato, CA: New World Library, 1999.

Byrne, Rhonda. *The Power*.
Great Britain: Simon & Schuster UK Ltd, 2010

Albers, Susan. *50 More Ways to Soothe Yourself Without Food: Mindfulness Strategies to Cope with Stress and End Emotional Eating*.
Canada: New Harbinger Publications, 2015

Lama, Dalai. *Many Ways to Nirvana: Reflections and Advice on Right Living*.
USA: Penguin Group, 2005

194

TRY SOMETHING DIFFERENT TODAY. DON'T STAY STUCK, DO BETTER.

ANDY WOOTEN